The EHRA Book of
Interventional Electrophysiology

Case-based learning with multiple choice questions

European Society of Cardiology publications

The ESC Textbook of Cardiovascular Medicine (Second Edition)
Edited by A. John Camm, Thomas F. Lüscher, and Patrick W. Serruys

The ESC Textbook of Intensive and Acute Cardiovascular Care (Second Edition)
Edited by Marco Tubaro, Pascal Vranckx, Susanna Price, and Christiaan Vrints

The ESC Textbook of Cardiovascular Imaging (Second Edition)
Edited by José Luis Zamorano, Jeroen Bax, Juhani Knuuti, Udo Sechtem, Patrizio Lancellotti, and Luigi Badano

The ESC Textbook of Preventive Cardiology
Edited by Stephan Gielen, Guy De Backer, Massimo F. Piepoli, and David Wood

The EHRA Book of Pacemaker, ICD, and CRT Troubleshooting: *Case-based learning with multiple choice questions*
Edited by Haran Burri, Carsten Israel, and Jean-Claude Deharo

The EACVI Echo Handbook
Edited by Patrizio Lancellotti and Bernard Cosyns

The ESC Handbook of Preventive Cardiology: *Putting prevention into practice*
Edited by Catriona Jennings, Ian Graham, and Stephan Gielen

The EACVI Textbook of Echocardiography (Second Edition)
Edited by Patrizio Lancellotti, José Luis Zamorano, Gilbert Habib, and Luigi Badano

The EHRA Book of Interventional Electrophysiology: *Case-based learning with multiple choice questions*
Edited by Hein Heidbuchel, Mattias Duytschaever, and Haran Burri

Forthcoming
The ESC Textbook of Vascular Biology
Edited by Robert Krams and Magnus Bäck

The ESC Textbook of Cardiovascular Development
Edited by Jose Maria Perez Pomares and Robert Kelly

The EHRA Book of

Interventional Electrophysiology

Case-based learning with multiple choice questions

Edited by

Hein Heidbuchel
University of Antwerp and University
Hospital Antwerp, Antwerp, Belgium

Mattias Duytschaever
Sint-Jan Hospital Bruges, Department of
Cardiology, Bruges, Belgium

Haran Burri
Cardiology Department, University
Hospital of Geneva, Switzerland

OXFORD
UNIVERSITY PRESS

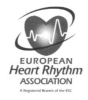

EUROPEAN
Heart Rhythm
ASSOCIATION
A Registered Branch of the ESC

EUROPEAN
SOCIETY OF
CARDIOLOGY®

UNIVERSITY PRESS

Great Clarendon Street, Oxford, OX2 6DP,
United Kingdom

Oxford University Press is a department of the University of Oxford.
It furthers the University's objective of excellence in research, scholarship,
and education by publishing worldwide. Oxford is a registered trade mark of
Oxford University Press in the UK and in certain other countries

Published in the United States of America by Oxford University Press
198 Madison Avenue, New York, NY 10016, United States of America

British Library Cataloguing in Publication Data
Data available

Library of Congress Control Number: 2016958221

ISBN 978-0-19-876637-7

Printed and bound by CPI Group (UK) Ltd, Croydon CR0 4YY

Endorsements

The basics of clinical cardiac electrophysiology set out with beautiful traces and clear concise explanations—an excellent and efficient learning resource.

John Camm
Professor of Clinical Cardiology,
St George's University of London,
London, UK

With great pleasure the European Heart Rhythm Association presents the first edition of *The EHRA Book of Interventional Electrophysiology*. This book closes a significant gap in the portfolio of EHRA educational products as it presents excellent clinical cases from interventional electrophysiology in a very practical fashion. All major fields of interventional electrophysiology are covered with interesting ECGs and EP tracings and beautifully illustrated clinical cases. In addition, the feature of self-assessment with multiple choice questions and the excellent comments and explanations complete the value of this educational tool. I would like to thank and congratulate the authors Hein Heidbuchel, Mattias Duytschaever and Haran Burri as well as all other case contributors for their excellent and outstanding work. This book is a 'must read' for everyone interested in clinical electrophysiology and will certainly contribute to improve the knowledge about heart rhythm disturbances and thereby the quality of care for the benefit of our patients with cardiac arrhythmias.

Gerhard Hindricks
EHRA President

The EHRA Book of Interventional Electrophysiology is a very enjoyable way to update yourself on all major types of recordings used in the EP laboratory. The cases are brief and to the point with very clear electrograms. They cover important electrogram observations, both common and uncommon. I recommend the text, and suspect that you will not want to put it down.

Warren M. (Sonny) Jackman, MD, FACC, FHRS
George Lynn Cross Research Professor of Medicine,
Heart Rhythm Institute,
University of Oklahoma Health Sciences Center,
Oklahoma City, USA

Preface

Our understanding of arrhythmias has evolved considerably over the years, as have the therapeutic options to treat our patients. Advances in mapping and ablation techniques have helped us tackle increasingly challenging cases in a faster, safer, and more effective manner. Despite these remarkable technological advances, it remains crucial that electrophysiologists fully understand fundamental principles that guide their procedures in the electrophysiology laboratory. In addition to theoretical knowledge, a keen sense of observation, and the ability to reason in a structured and logical manner are the keys to success.

Case-based learning is particularly well suited to test theoretical knowledge as well as to train the skills required of electrophysiologists. The cases presented in this book are a compilation of common and more unusual situations presented by sixteen experienced electrophysiologists. The tracings of the cases are each followed by a specific question, that is explained on a later page. The book is intentionally not divided into sections so as not to result in any bias when interpreting the tracings. The cases are of variable difficulty, but all cover essential principles that should be assimilated by the reader.

The material provided here will assist those studying for the European Heart Rhythm Association (EHRA) accreditation exam in electrophysiology. It is also intended to be read by more advanced practitioners who enjoy elucidating unknown tracings, and who appreciate that there is always something to learn.

We hope that you will enjoy going through the cases, and that the book will be of value for your clinical practice!

Hein Heidbuchel
Mattias Duytschaever
Haran Burri

Contents

Contributors

Jesus Almendral
(Cases 10 & 11)

Haran Burri
(Cases 4, 19, 25, 26, 44, 45, & 73)

Jacques De Bakker
(Cases 9, 18, 24, 43, & 50)

Thomas Deneke
(Cases 23, 33, 34, 42, 69, & 74)

Mattias Duytschaever & Rene Tavernier
(Cases 1, 17, 20, 21, 27, 35, 36, 41, 51, 52, 61, 68, 72, 75, & 76)

Hein Heidbuchel
(Cases 2, 5, 6, 7, 15, 16, 29, 38, 39, 62, 63, 67, 70, & 71)

Josef Kautzner
(Cases 49, 54, 55, & 60)

Pier Lambiase
(3, 28, 30, & 53)

Maurizio Lunati
(Cases 22, 31, 32, 65, & 66)

Robert Pap
(Cases 8, 12, 56, & 64)

Stefano Pedretti
(Cases 22, 31, 32, 65, & 66)

Petr Peichl
(Cases 49, 54, 55, & 60)

Frédéric Sacher
(Cases 46, 47, 48, 58, & 59)

Laszlo Saghy
(Cases 8, 12, 56, & 64)

Christoph Scharf
(Cases 13, 14, 37, 40, & 57)

Cristina Tutuianu
(Cases 8, 12, 56, & 64)

Symbols and abbreviations

°C	degree Celsius
δ	delta
Δ	delta
=	equal to
≥	equal to or greater than
≤	equal to or less than
<	less than
>	more than
Ω	ohm
%	per cent
±	plus or minus
AH	atrio-His (interval)
APD	action potential duration
ARI	activation recovery interval
ARVC	arrhythmogenic right ventricular cardiomyopathy
AT	atrial tachycardia
AV	atrioventricular
AVNRT	atrioventricular nodal re-entrant tachycardia
AVRT	atrioventricular re-entrant tachycardia
BBRVT	bundle branch re-entrant ventricular tachycardia
bpm	beat per minute
CRT-D	cardiac resynchronization therapy defibrillator
CS	coronary sinus
CTI	cavo-tricuspid isthmus
DCM	dilated cardiomyopathy
ECG	electrocardiogram
HA	His-to-atrium
Hz	hertz

ICD	implantable cardioverter–defibrillator
JET	junctional ectopic tachycardia
LAO	left anterior oblique
LAVA	local abnormal ventricular activity
LBB	left bundle branch
LBBB	left bundle branch block
LCP	lower common pathway
LSPV	left superior pulmonary vein
LV	left ventricle/ventricular
LVEF	left ventricular ejection fraction
LVOT	left ventricular outflow tract
mA	milliampere
MI	myocardial infarction
min	minute
mm	millimetre
ms	millisecond
mV	millivolt
NYHA	New York Heart Association
ORT	orthodromic reciprocating tachycardia
PAC	premature atrial complex
PJRT	permanent junctional reciprocating tachycardia
PPI	post-pacing interval
PV	pulmonary vein
PVC	premature ventricular contraction/complexes
PVI	pulmonary vein isolation
RAO	right anterior oblique
RIPV	right inferior pulmonary vein
RSPV	right superior pulmonary vein

RV	right ventricular/ventricle
RVOT	right ventricular outflow tract
s	second
SA	sinoatrial
SVC	superior vena cava
SVT	supraventricular tachycardia
TCL	tachycardia cycle length
VA	ventriculoatrial
VF	ventricular fibrillation
VPC	ventricular premature complex
VT	ventricular tachycardia
W	watt

Introduction to the case

This case presents a 44-year-old carpenter with transient left bundle branch (LBBB) morphology during tachycardia (Figure 1.1).

Figure 1.1 Surface leads II, aVR, aVF, V1, and V5, and intracardiac recordings from the distal His bundle (HB), coronary sinus (CS), and right ventricular (RV) base

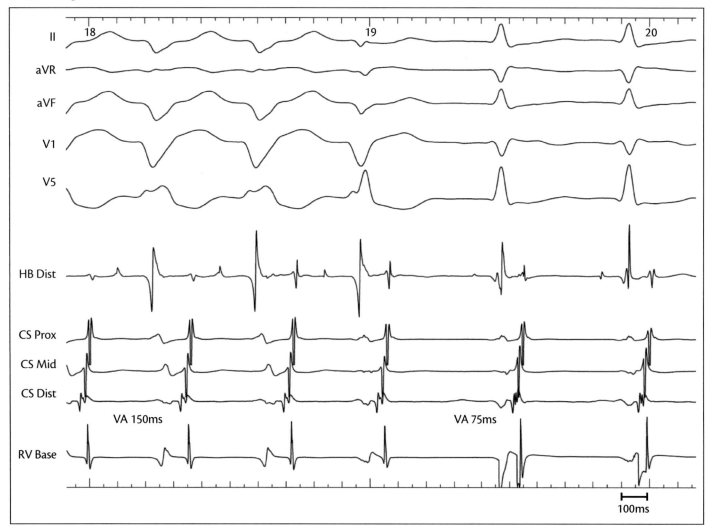

Question

In this tracing, transient left bundle branch block (LBBB) is associated with a change in tachycardia cycle length. Which statement is true regarding this tracing?

A Cycle length prolongs during LBBB because of an ipsilateral accessory pathway

B Cycle length prolongs during LBBB because of a contralateral accessory pathway

C Cycle length prolongs and infra-His conduction resumes because of a shift to antero-grade slow pathway conduction

D Cycle length prolongs and infra-His conduction resumes due to slowing of a left-sided ectopic atrial tachycardia (AT)

E Cycle length prolongs and infra-His conduction 'resumes' due to anterograde block over a Mahaim fibre

Answer

C   **Cycle length prolongs and infra-His conduction resumes because of a shift to anterograde slow pathway conduction**

Explanation

Orthodromic atrioventricular re-entrant tachycardia using dual anterograde nodal conduction

The underlying mechanism is orthodromic atrioventricular re-entrant tachycardia (AVRT) (anterograde nodal conduction, retrograde via left-sided bypass tract). Conventionally, LBBB during orthodromic AVRT over a left-sided bypass tract usually is associated with prolongation of the atrial cycle length (due to the larger circuit).

In the present case, the shorter cycle length during LBBB is somewhat paradoxical ('accelerating LBBB') and needs explaining. In the left part, rate-dependent LBB aberrancy is present. Most likely, LBB aberrancy perpetuates via concealed trans-septal retrograde conduction until this phenomenon is interrupted by retrograde invasion of a left-sided premature ventricular complex (PVC) into the left bundle. Moreover, this His-refractory PVC resets the atrium (excluding AT and proving active participation of the bypass tract). The resulting shorter A–A interval causes a shift in anterograde conduction from the fast to the slow pathway. Together with peeling back refractoriness of the left bundle, cycle length prolongation results in normal infra-Hisian conduction. After ablation of the left-sided bypass tract, the patient was not inducible for atrioventricular nodal re-entrant tachycardia (AVNRT).

Note: In this setting, measurement of the ventriculoatrial (VA) interval from QRS onset to the earliest atrial electrogram, instead of the cycle length, is less ambiguous. VA prolongation of >40ms provides strong evidence of a free wall accessory pathway in ipsilateral bundle branch block in the absence of a pre-existing underlying fascicular block.

Introduction to the case

Case 2 focuses on a woman, aged 33, with paroxysmal palpitations (no electrocardiogram (ECG)). During an electrophysiological study, this tracing was recorded during incremental atrial pacing (Figure 2.1).

Figure 2.1 Intracardiac electrograms during pacing from the right atrial appendage at a cycle length of 360ms. RAA: right atrial appendage; HBp till HBd: His bundle recordings from proximal to distal; RV: right ventricle; S: stimulus; H: His bundle deflection.

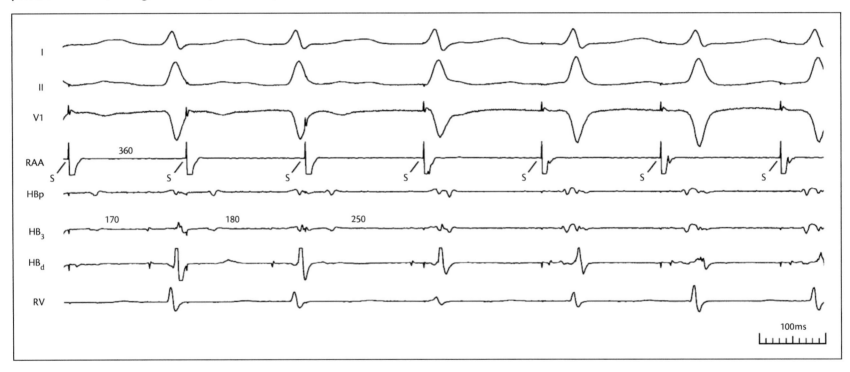

Question

The tracing shows:

A   A jump from fast to slow pathway, with 1-to-1 antegrade conduction over the slow pathway. This is a hallmark of AVNRT

B   A jump from fast to slow pathway as can be seen in any patient—aspecific

C   Conduction over a Mahaim-type accessory pathway

D   Conduction over a regular-type accessory pathway

E   Atrioventricular (AV) dissociation

Answer

A   **A jump from fast to slow pathway, with 1-to-1 antegrade conduction over the slow pathway. This is a hallmark of AVNRT**

Explanation

Atrioventricular conduction during incremental pacing

Atrial pacing at a cycle length of 360ms leads to a rapidly progressive atrio-His (AH) prolongation with a sudden increase of ≥50ms and with stabilization later on at a value of >220ms (which is often seen as the maximal AH interval for conduction over the fast pathway). From beat 3 on, there is therefore 1-to-1 conduction over the slow pathway. While many patients show a jump to the slow pathway during incremental atrial pacing, this usually prolongs further during the ensuing beats and is followed by AV block (i.e. a Wenckebach sequence). The 1-to-1 conduction is often seen in patients with AVNRT (using the slow pathway for antegrade conduction), since for the arrhythmia to sustain, every beat needs to be conducted over the slow pathway.[1] Elimination of 1-to-1 conduction over the slow pathway is also an indirect endpoint for successful AVNRT ablation, apart from non-inducibility.

References

1. Jackman WM, Beckman KJ, McClelland JH, *et al.* Treatment of supraventricular tachycardia due to atrioventricular nodal reentry, by radiofrequency catheter ablation of slow-pathway conduction. *N Engl J Med* 1992; **327**: 313–18.

Introduction to the case

Case 3 is regarding a 35-year-old woman with a history of recurrent palpitations. She had no prior history of syncope and has a structurally normal heart on echocardiography. A 4-wire electrophysiological study was performed and during an antegrade curve (S1 400ms, S2 260ms), the following tachycardia was induced (Figure 3.1). The VA intervals are outlined on the coronary sinus (CS) channel. During tachycardia, the following phenomenon is observed.

Figure 3.1 Surface leads I, aVF, V1, and V4, and intracardiac recordings from the distal and proximal bipoles of the His bundle (His), the proximal to distal bipoles of the coronary sinus (CS), and the right ventricular apex (RV)

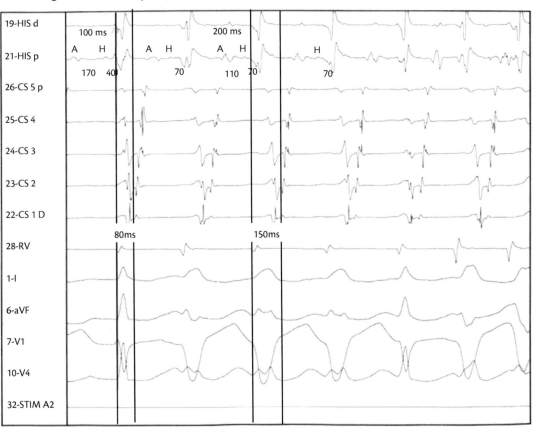

Question

What is the mechanism of tachycardia?

A   AVNRT with intermittent bundle branch block

B   AVRT with intermittent pre-excitation

C   AT with intermittent LBBB

D   Orthodromic AVRT using a left lateral pathway

E   AT with intermittent pre-excitation

Answer

D   Orthodromic AVRT using a left lateral pathway

Explanation

Narrow versus wide QRS during tachycardia

This tracing demonstrates an eccentric atrial activation sequence which would be consistent with a left AT or the presence of a left lateral accessory pathway. There is one diagnostic feature which proves that the left lateral accessory pathway is a critical part of the circuit—there is intermittent LBBB with VA prolongation during the LBBB beats. This phenomenon of VA prolongation during orthodromic tachycardia using an accessory pathway ipsilateral to the bundle branch block was originally described by Coumel. Often it prolongs the tachycardia cycle length (TCL) as the re-entrant wavefront is forced to take a longer route via the contralateral bundle branch (right bundle in this case). However, the cycle length may remain the same despite ipsilateral bundle branch block if the AH interval shortens to compensate (or, in other words, no cycle length prolongation does not exclude an ipsilateral accessory pathway). Hence, it is crucial to measure the VA interval (from the onset of the QRS complex to the earliest atrial electrogram) to make the diagnosis, and not just the TCL.[1] VA prolongation by ≥40ms provides strong evidence of a free wall AP in ipsilateral bundle branch block in the absence of a pre-existing underlying fascicular block.

References

1. Yang Y, Cheng J, Glatter K, Dorostkar P, Modin GW, Scheinman MM. Quantitative effects of functional bundle branch block in patients with atrioventricular reentrant tachycardia. *Am J Cardiol* 2000; **85**: 826–31.

Introduction to the case

A 68-year-old patient with pre-existent LBBB underwent an electrophysiological study for syncope. During placement of a catheter in the right ventricle (RV), asystole during 4s occurred with resumption of a rhythm, as shown in Figure 4.1a. The quadripolar catheter was retracted to the His bundle region, revealing the recording shown in Figure 4.1b.

Figure 4.1 Asystole during 4s occurred with resumption of a rhythm, as shown in (a). The quadripolar catheter was retracted to the His bundle region, revealing the recording shown in (b). His d, distal His; His p, proximal His

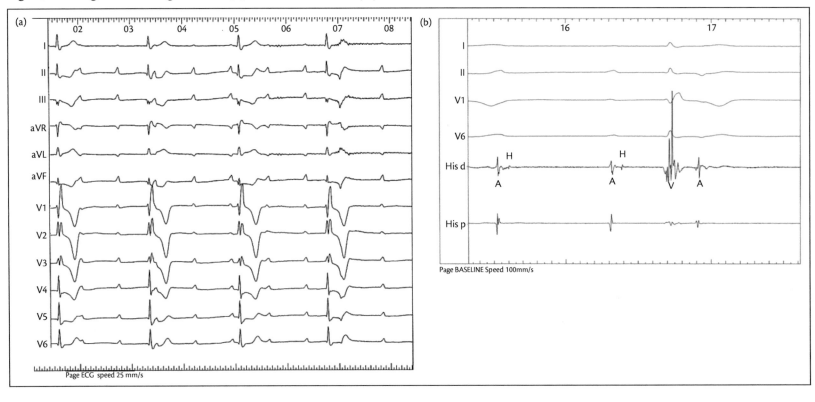

Question

What do you observe?

A   Third-degree AV block (supra-Hisian)

B   Second-degree AV block

C   Infra-Hisian block with complete dissociation

D   Infra-Hisian unidirectional block

E   Intra-Hisian conduction delay

Answer

D Infra-Hisian unidirectional block

Explanation

Infra-Hisian complete atrioventricular block with VA conduction

The tracings show infra-Hisian antegrade AV block, with a ventricular escape rhythm probably originating from a left septal fascicle (judging by the typical right bundle branch block pattern). The last cycle of this ventricular escape rhythm is followed by an early atrial event with negative P-wave morphology in lead II, compatible with retrograde conduction, indicating preserved VA conduction. The other QRS complexes are not followed by a retrograde P-wave, due to closely spaced sinus P-waves rendering the atrium refractory. It is impossible to ascertain whether there is intra-Hisian conduction delay, as a His deflection is not visible on the proximal His recording, but the fact that the block occurred during placement of the right ventricular catheter is strongly suggestive of traumatic right bundle branch block. This case illustrates how care should be taken when placing the RV catheter in patients with an underlying LBBB (which was thus shown to be indeed complete in our patient), due to the risk of traumatic right bundle branch block with resulting complete heart block. AV conduction resumed in our patient after 10 minutes, and a pacemaker was implanted under the assumption that syncope had occurred due to paroxysmal complete AV block.

Introduction to the case

Case 5 studies a man, aged 42 years, who had an electrophysiological study for paroxysmal supraventricular tachycardia. At the beginning of the study, pacing is performed from the distal His bundle electrode, while the output of the pacing impulse is switched between 20mA (@ 2ms; left side of the tracing) and 2mA (right side of the tracing) (Figure 5.1). What diagnostic information can be retrieved from the tracing?

Figure 5.1 The output of the pacing impulse is switched between 20mA (@ 2ms; left side of the tracing) and 2mA (right side of the tracing). RAA: right atrial appendage; HBp till HBd: His bundle recordings from proximal to distal; PS: posteroseptal position (between tricuspid annulus and coronary sinus ostium); CS: coronary sinus; S: stimulus

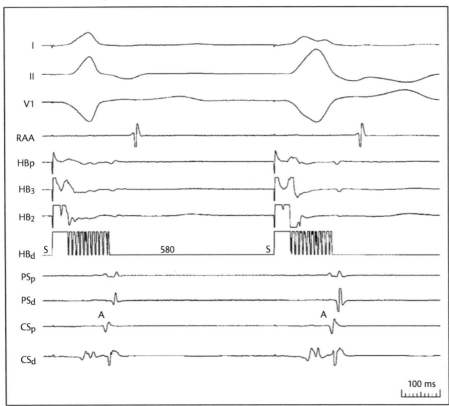

Question

The information from the tracing is:

A   Nothing relevant

B   That the patient has atrial tachycardia

C   That the patient has retrograde conduction over the fast pathway

D   That the patient had retrograde conduction over the slow pathway

E   That the patient has retrograde conduction over an accessory pathway

Answer

E **That the patient has retrograde conduction over an accessory pathway**

Explanation

Para-Hisian pacing/1

It can be readily observed that the QRS complex on the left side is narrower than that on the right side (Figure 5.2). While pacing at a high output, not only is the ventricular septum captured, but the distal right bundle itself also is.[1,2] Therefore, part of the ventricles is activated via the His–Purkinje system, explaining the narrower QRS. In the electrograms on the right side, a retrograde His bundle deflection can be appreciated after the local ventricular electrogram in the His bundle electrodes, due to the fact that only the ventricular myocardium is captured with the low output of 2mA. Since the ventricular activation has to proceed first to the apex before it can enter the Purkinje system and conduct retrogradely, the activation of the proximal His bundle (which is the input to the AV node) is delayed; while the S–S interval is 580ms, the interval between consecutive proximal His bundle activations is 635ms. Nevertheless, the interval between both atrial activation sequences (which are identical in both beats, with first atrial activation at the proximal CS catheter) is nearly the same as the pacing interval (585ms). This can only be explained if atrial activation is not dependent on His bundle activation, i.e. when it is not proceeding over the AV node. Retrograde conduction is proceeding over a direct connection between the ventricle and atrium, i.e. an accessory pathway, since the timing of ventricular activation at the base of the ventricles is identical in both paced beats (Figure 5.3). The slight delay in atrial activation is due to the fact that ventricular activation at the insertion of the accessory pathway may be reached slightly faster in case the His–Purkinje system is involved in ventricular activation as in the left-sided beat. Earliest atrial activation points to a posteroseptal accessory pathway (concealed or overt, which cannot be distinguished from this tracing).

Figure 5.2 Same figure as Figure 5.1, but now including annotations on timing, electrograms, and the tissues being captured in the 1st and 2nd beats.

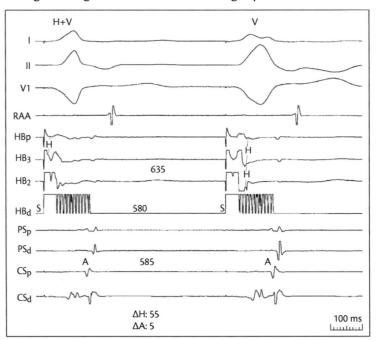

Figure 5.3 (a) Capture of the His bundle/proximal right bundle and local ventricular myocardium. (b) Capture of only the local ventricular myocardium

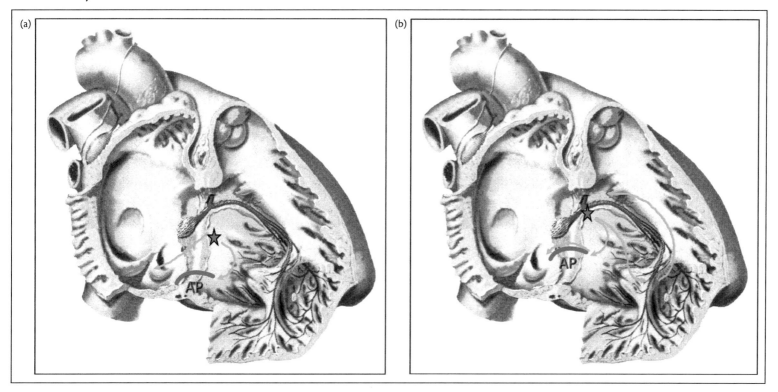

References

1. Hirao K, Otomo K, Wang X, *et al*. Para-Hisian pacing: a new method for differentiating retrograde conduction over an accessory AV pathway from conduction over the AV node. *Circulation* 1996; **94**: 1027–35.

2. Heidbuchel H, Ector H, Adams J, Van de Werf F. Use of only a regular diagnostic His-bundle catheter for both fast and reproducible "para-Hisian pacing" and stable right ventricular pacing. *J Cardiovasc Electrophysiol* 1997; **8**: 1121–32.

Introduction to the case

Case 6 discusses a woman, aged 18, regarding an electrophysiological study for paroxysmal supraventricular tachycardia. At the beginning of the study, pacing is performed from the distal His bundle electrode, while the output of the pacing impulse is switched between 20mA (@ 2ms; left side of the tracing) and 2mA (right side of the tracing) (Figure 6.1). What diagnostic information can be retrieved from the tracing?

Figure 6.1 The left panel shows a sinus beat. In the right panel, pacing is performed from the distal His bundle electrode, while the output of the pacing impulse is switched between 20mA (@ 2ms; left side of the tracing) and 2mA (right side of the tracing). RAA: right atrial appendage; HBp till HBd: His bundle recordings from proximal to distal; PS: posteroseptal position (between the tricuspid annulus and coronary sinus ostium); CS: coronary sinus; S: stimulus

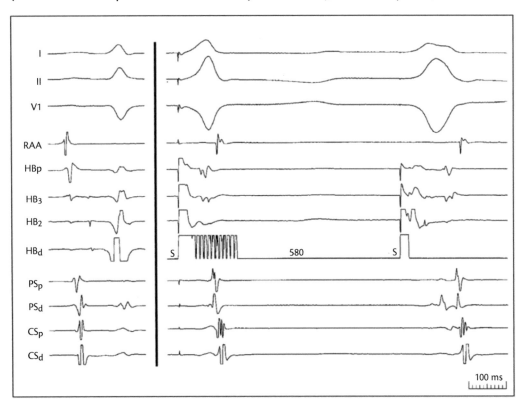

Question

The information from the tracing is:

A   Nothing relevant

B   That the patient has atrial tachycardia

C   That the patient has retrograde conduction over the fast pathway

D   That the patient has retrograde conduction over the slow pathway

E   That the patient has retrograde conduction over an accessory pathway

Answer

C **That the patient has retrograde conduction over the fast pathway**

Explanation

Para-Hisian pacing/2

This is another example of para-Hisian pacing with a narrower QRS complex on the left side and a wider one on the right side, due to capture of both the right bundle and the ventricular myocardium, respectively, of only the ventricular myocardium (Figure 6.2).[1,2] Again, the timing of retrograde His bundle activation is changed, appreciable in the proximal His bundle electrodes. In this case, however: (1) earliest retrograde atrial activation is occurring at the anterior septum (apparent from the His bundle electrodes), and (2) the timing of the whole atrial activation is delayed just as much as the His bundle timing is delayed. This indicates that this retrograde activation is occurring over the fast AV nodal pathway. While this proves that the observed activation is occurring over the fast AV nodal pathway, this does not 100% exclude the presence of a concealed accessory pathway. Especially for accessory pathways with a long retrograde conduction time or that are located far from the stimulation site (e.g. left lateral), conduction of the fast pathway may still be faster than conduction over the accessory pathway, even with a delay in His bundle activation as in the beats without His bundle capture.

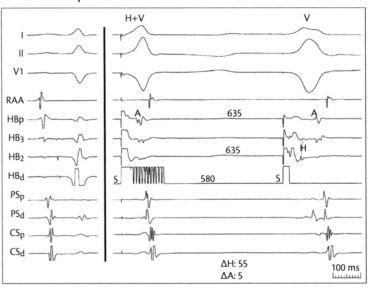

Figure 6.2 Same figure as Figure 6.1, but with extra annotations and timings. See text for explanation.

References

1. Hirao K, Otomo K, Wang X, *et al.* Para-Hisian pacing: a new method for differentiating retrograde conduction over an accessory AV pathway from conduction over the AV node. *Circulation* 1996; **94**: 1027–35.

2. Heidbuchel H, Ector H, Adams J, Van de Werf F. Use of only a regular diagnostic His-bundle catheter for both fast and reproducible 'para-Hisian pacing' and stable right ventricular pacing. *J Cardiovasc Electrophysiol* 1997; **8**: 1121–32.

Introduction to the case

A woman, aged 28, with an electrophysiological study for paroxysmal supraventricular tachycardia is the focus for Case 7. At the beginning of the study, pacing is performed from the distal His bundle electrode, while the output of the pacing impulse is switched between 20mA (@ 2ms; left side of the tracing) and 2mA (right side of the tracing) (Figure 7.1). What diagnostic information can be retrieved from the tracing?

Figure 7.1 Paroxysmal supraventricular tachycardia. RAA: right atrial appendage; HBp till HBd: His bundle recordings from proximal to distal; CS: coronary sinus; S: stimulus

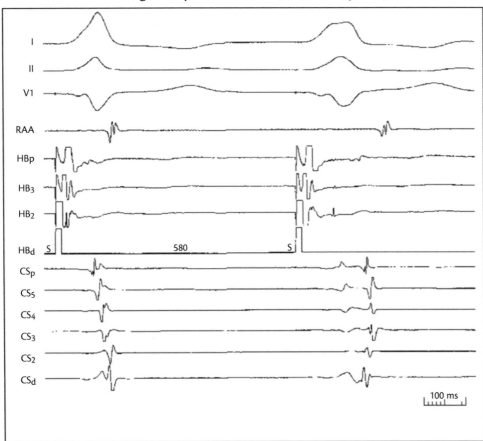

Question

The information from the tracing is:

A That the patient has retrograde conduction over the fast pathway

B That the patient has retrograde conduction over the slow pathway

C That the patient has retrograde conduction over an accessory pathway

D That the patient has retrograde conduction over an accessory pathway and the fast pathway

E That the patient has retrograde conduction over an accessory pathway and the slow pathway

Answer

D **That the patient has retrograde conduction over an accessory pathway and the fast pathway**

Explanation

Para-Hisian pacing/3

Again this is an example of para-Hisian pacing.[1,2] In contrast to the two previous examples, the retrograde atrial activation is not the same during both beats (Figure 7.2). This indicates that there must be some form of fusion explaining one or both beats of the tracing. A close look at the timing of retrograde His bundle activation and those of the atrial electrograms at different locations shows that the anteroseptal atrial electrogram 'moves out' with the same amount as the proximal His bundle itself, indicating that it depends on His bundle input and thus is due to nodal conduction. In contrast, the electrogram in the distal CS moves out much less when His bundle capture is lost (and His bundle activation is delayed) in the right beat. This proves that it does not depend on His bundle timing and is due to conduction over an accessory pathway. As explained earlier, the A–A interval in the CS (where the left-sided accessory pathway is located) is somewhat longer than the H–H interval, which is due to faster left lateral ventricular activation when the His bundle is captured (in the beat on the left), and the His–Purkinje system helps swifter activation of the left ventricular (LV) lateral wall.

References

1. Hirao K, Otomo K, Wang X, *et al.* Para-Hisian pacing: a new method for differentiating retrograde conduction over an accessory AV pathway from conduction over the AV node. *Circulation* 1996; **94**: 1027–35.

2. Heidbuchel H, Ector H, Adams J, Van de Werf F. Use of only a regular diagnostic His-bundle catheter for both fast and reproducible "para-Hisian pacing" and stable right ventricular pacing. *J Cardiovasc Electrophysiol* 1997; **8**: 1121–32.

Figure 7.2 Same figure as Figure 7.1, but now including annotations on timing, electrograms, and the tissues being captured in the 1st and 2nd beats.

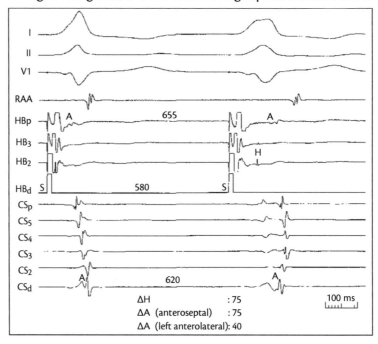

Introduction to the case

Case 8 discusses a woman who is 58 years old, presenting with regular palpitations and documented narrow QRS complex tachycardia. During an electrophysiological study, a sustained tachycardia with a cycle length of 380ms with a long VA interval (277ms) was induced. Overdrive ventricular pacing was performed and the following result was obtained reproducibly (Figure 8.1).

Figure 8.1 Regular palpitations and documented narrow QRS complex tachycardia. CS 9, 10: proximal coronary sinus; CS 5, 6: middle coronary sinus; CS 1, 2: distal coronary sinus; RVA: right ventricular apex; His d: distal bipole of His catheter; His p: proximal bipole of His catheter

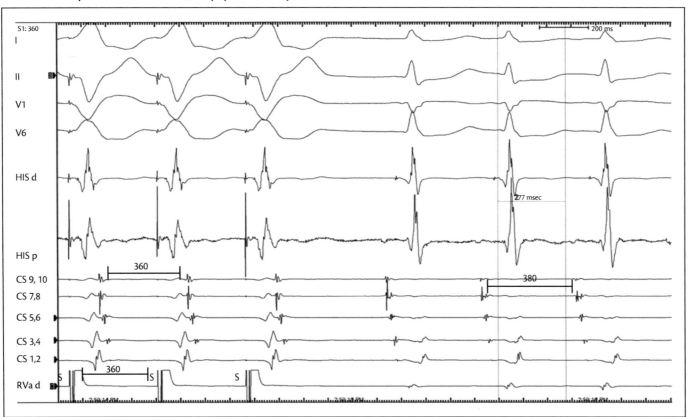

Question

The response of this pacing manoeuvre is suggestive that the mechanism of the tachycardia is:

A Atrial tachycardia

B Typical AVNRT

C Atypical AVNRT

D AVRT using a concealed accessory pathway

E The tachycardia was not entrained

Answer

A   Atrial tachycardia

Explanation

Ventricular overdrive pacing during supraventricular tachycardia

Entrainment of the tachycardia by ventricular pacing (the atrial cycle length was accelerated to the pacing cycle length, and the tachycardia continues after pacing was stopped) reveals a VAAV response, following cessation of overdrive ventricular pacing, and is typical for the diagnosis of AT.[1,2]

References

1. Veenhuyzen GD, Quinn FR, Wilton SB, Clegg R, Mitchell LB. Diagnostic pacing maneuvers for supraventricular tachycardia: part 1. *Pacing Clin Electrophysiol* 2011; **34**: 767–82.

2. Josephson ME (2002). *Clinical Cardiac Electrophysiology*, 3rd edn. Philadelphia: Lippincott, Williams, & Wilkins.

Introduction to the case

The configuration of the unipolar electrogram (Figure 9.1) provides information about the movement of the activation front at the recording site. At the site where activation arises, the unipolar electrogram only has a negative deflection. If the activation front is passing the recording site, the unipolar electrogram is biphasic, whereas the configuration is only positive at a site where activation comes to an end.

Figure 9.1 Configuration of the unipolar electrogram

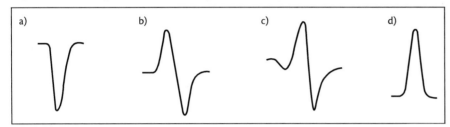

Question

Which configuration of the unipolar electrograms shown in the figure occurs at the 'origin' (exit site) of an infarct-related re-entrant tachycardia?

A   A negative deflection only

B   A biphasic deflection

C   A biphasic deflection with a small initial negative component

D   A positive deflection only

Answer

A A negative deflection only

Explanation

Unipolar electrogram morphology

In the unipolar electrogram, a positive deflection is generated by the approaching wavefront, whereas the receding wavefront produces a negative deflection.[1] Infarct-related tachycardias are usually based on re-entry where the re-entrant circuit consists of small surviving myocardial bundles in the infarcted zone and remaining healthy myocardium (Figure 9.2). Because at all recording sites along a re-entrant circuit the wavefront is passing, a biphasic deflection would be expected to occur at all sites. The site where activation in the surviving bundle within the infarction leaves the infarcted zone and activates the remaining healthy myocardium is the exit site. Because the diameter of the myocardial bundle is usually very small, the positive deflection of the approaching wavefront is virtually missing (the few myocardial cells in the bundle generate hardly any current). Only the large receding wavefront in the adjacent healthy myocardium generates a large negative deflection.[2–4]

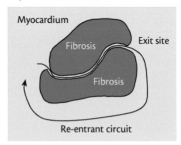

Figure 9.2 Depiction of re-entrant circuit within the myocardial scar

References

1. de Bakker JMT, Hauer RNW, Simmers TA (1995). Activation mapping: unipolar versus bipolar recording. In: DP Zipes, J Jalife (eds.). *Cardiac Electrophysiology: From Cell to Bedside*, 2nd edn. Philadelphia: WB Saunders Company, pp. 1068–78.

2. Durrer D, Formijne P, van Dam R, van Lier A, Buller J, Meyler FL. The electrocardiogram in normal and some abnormal conditions in revived human fetal heart and in acute and chronic coronary occlusion. *Am Heart J* 1961; **61**: 303–16.

3. Spach MS, Barr RC, Johnson EA, Kootsey JM. Cardiac extracellular potentials: analysis of complex wave forms about the Purkinje networks in dogs. *Circ Res* 1973; **33**: 465–73.

4. Stevenson WG, Soejima K. Recording techniques for clinical electrophysiology. *J Cardiovasc Electrophysiol* 2005; **16**: 1017–22.

Introduction to the case

This case presents a 67-year-old with documented wide QRS complex tachycardia. During the electrophysiological study, a wide QRS complex regular tachycardia was reproducibly induced (Figure 10.1). The tachycardia had an LBBB morphology, with 1:1 VA relationship, an HV interval of 55ms, and an eccentric atrial activation, all consistent with a left free wall accessory pathway-mediated tachycardia. However, look at the response to continuous ventricular pacing during tachycardia. An RV pacing train (cycle length 410) was delivered during tachycardia. The end of the pacing train is showed, followed by continuation of the tachycardia.

Figure 10.1 Wide QRS complex tachycardia. CS, coronary sinus; RV, right ventricle; SA, interval from stimulus to atrial electrogram; VA, interval from QRS onset to atrial electrogram

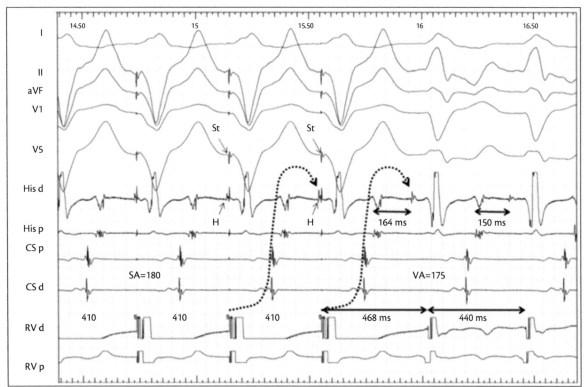

Question

The tracing shows an orthodromic tachycardia mediated by a left-sided accessory pathway. The QRS displays LBBB. What can be considered unexpected in this tracing?

A   The atrial activation sequence during pacing and that during tachycardia are identical

B   The His bundle electrogram is antegrade during ventricular pacing

C   The AH during ventricular pacing is longer than that during tachycardia

D   The stimulus-A (SA) interval and the VA interval are almost identical

E   All the above are unexpected

Answer

D **The stimulus-A (SA) interval and the VA interval are almost identical**

Explanation

Entrainment of orthodromic atrioventricular re-entrant tachycardia by right ventricular pacing in the presence of left bundle branch block

The tracing shows that ventricular pacing at a constant rate produces transient entrainment of the tachycardia. For that to be the case, each paced ventricular wavefront is colliding with the antegrade wavefront propagating through the AV conducting system, probably at the level of the right bundle branch. In such a scenario, atrial activation occurs exclusively via the accessory pathway, so its activation sequence should be identical as that during tachycardia. The His bundle is activated by the descending wavefront of the tachycardia, so it is an antegrade His. As a consequence, the AH interval is similar as that during tachycardia, but usually a bit longer since the pacing rate is faster than the tachycardia rate. It has been observed that, in orthodromic tachycardias mediated by left-sided accessory pathways, the SA interval is longer than the VA interval (mean difference in the range of 70ms), although the difference is less than in AV nodal re-entry.[1,2] So almost identical SA and VA intervals are unexpected. The explanation for this unexpected finding in this case is that the SA interval normally exceeds the VA interval because pacing occurs at a distance from the pathway (RV pacing, left-sided pathway), but in this case the circuit has become bigger due to the LBBB, so the RV pacing site is close to the re-entrant circuit.

References

1. Almendral J. Resetting and entrainment of reentrant arrhythmias: part II: informative content and practical use of these responses. *Pacing Clin Electrophysiol* 2013; **36**: 641–61.

2. González-Torrecilla E, Almendral J, García-Fernández FJ, *et al*. Differences in ventriculoatrial intervals during entrainment and tachycardia: a simpler method for distinguishing paroxysmal supraventricular tachycardia with long ventriculoatrial intervals. *J Cardiovasc Electrophysiol* 2011; **22**: 915–21.

Introduction to the case

A 44-year-old man with recurrent episodes of tachycardia in the absence of structural heart disease underwent an electrophysiological evaluation. A regular, sustained narrow QRS tachycardia was induced at a cycle length of 420ms. However, RV extrastimuli, despite advancing the atrium, could not be proven to do so during a refractory His. In the electrophysiology lab, as in real life, any unexpected event should be looked at (Figure 11.1). Can a spontaneous ventricular premature complex (VPC) that occurred during tachycardia help?

Figure 11.1 Documented regular narrow QRS tachycardias. ABLA, ablation catheter located at the AV junction; HRA, high right atrium; VD, right ventricle

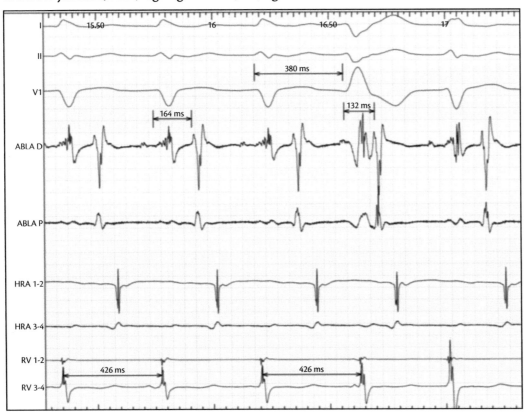

Question

What is the most likely mechanism of this tachycardia?

A   AV nodal re-entry

B   Orthodromic, mediated by a right-sided accessory pathway

C   Orthodromic, mediated by a left-sided accessory pathway

D   Orthodromic, but there is no clue as to the location of the accessory pathway

E   The tracing is not conclusive, since not all ventricular tissue is captured by the VPC: the RV electrogram is not advanced

Answer

C   **Orthodromic, mediated by a left-sided accessory pathway**

Explanation

Atrial reset by a ventricular fusion beat during orthodromic atrioventricular re-entrant tachycardia and importance of ventricular premature beat location

The VPC clearly advances the atria without advancing the His bundle recording, establishing the presence of an accessory pathway. The fact that the RV electrogram is not advanced at the time of the VPC is actually important because it establishes that there is ventricular fusion. Advancing the atria by a ventricular depolarization with fusion provides further evidence of the presence of an accessory pathway.[1] It has been reported that RV stimulation with fused beats can advance the atria during orthodromic tachycardia in the presence of septal or right-sided accessory pathways (pacing close to their ventricular insertion), but not in the presence of left-sided accessory pathways.[2] It has also been reported that LV pacing produces entrainment with fusion of orthodromic tachycardias mediated by left-sided accessory pathways. In this tracing, the VPC has a right bundle configuration (and is negative in lead I), presumably coming from the LV and producing resetting with fusion, so it is more likely that the accessory pathway is left-sided.

References

1. Ormaetxe JM, Almendral J, Arenal A, *et al*. Ventricular fusion during resetting and entrainment of orthodromic supraventricular tachycardia involving septal accessory pathways. Implications for the differential diagnosis with atrioventricular nodal reentry. *Circulation* 1993; **88**: 2623–31.

2. Suyama K, Ohe T, Kurita T, *et al*. Significance of ventricular pacing site in manifest entrainment during orthodromic atrioventricular reentrant tachycardia with left-sided accessory pathway. *Pacing Clin Electrophysiol* 1992; **15**: 1114–21.

Introduction to the case

A 32-year-old man is presented with recurrent palpitations and documented narrow QRS tachycardia. During an electrophysiological study, after induction of the tachycardia, the introduction of a PVC during His refractoriness was performed, and the result was consequently reproducible (Figure 12.1).

Figure 12.1 PVC during His refractoriness. CS 9, 10: proximal coronary sinus; CS 5, 6: middle coronary sinus; CS 1, 2: distal coronary sinus; H: His electrogram; His d, distal; His p, proximal bipoles of a catheter in the His region; RVA, right ventricular apex; S, stimulation artefact

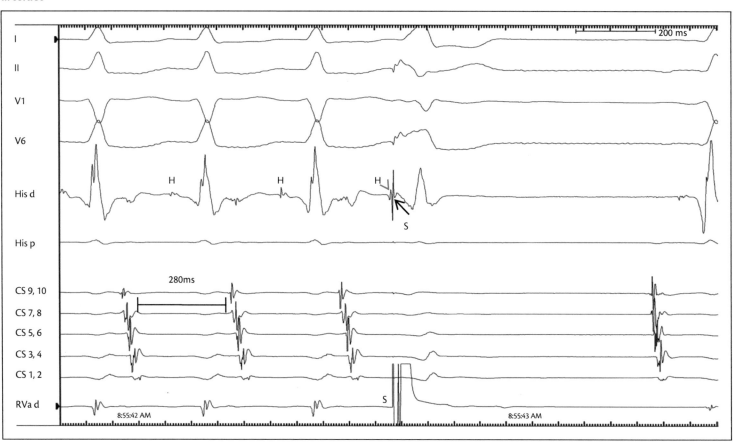

Question

What is most likely mechanism of the tachycardia?

A   Typical AVNRT

B   Atypical AVNRT

C   AVRT using an accessory pathway

D   Atrial tachycardia

E   There are not enough data

Answer

C **AVRT using an accessory pathway**

Explanation

A single ventricular extrastimulus during supraventricular tachycardia/1

The tachycardia is a narrow complex supraventricular tachycardia. The fact that the PVC during His refractoriness terminates the tachycardia without conduction to the atrium indicates that an accessory pathway is present and is participating in the re-entry circuit. This cannot be the case in AT or AVNRT, not even over a bystander pathway.[1,2]

References

1. Veenhuyzen GD, Quinn FR, Wilton SB, Clegg R, Mitchell LB. Diagnostic pacing maneuvers for supraventricular tachycardias: part 2. *Pacing Clin Electrophysiol* 2012; **35**: 757–69.

2. Huang SKS, Wood MA (2011). *Catheter Ablation of Cardiac Arrhythmias*, 2nd edn. Philadelphia: Elsevier Saunders.

Introduction to the case

During atrial pacing, the following tachycardia is induced (Figure 13.1).

Figure 13.1 Top surface ECG lead I, aVF, V1, and V6. HRA, high right atrium; RVA, right ventricular apex

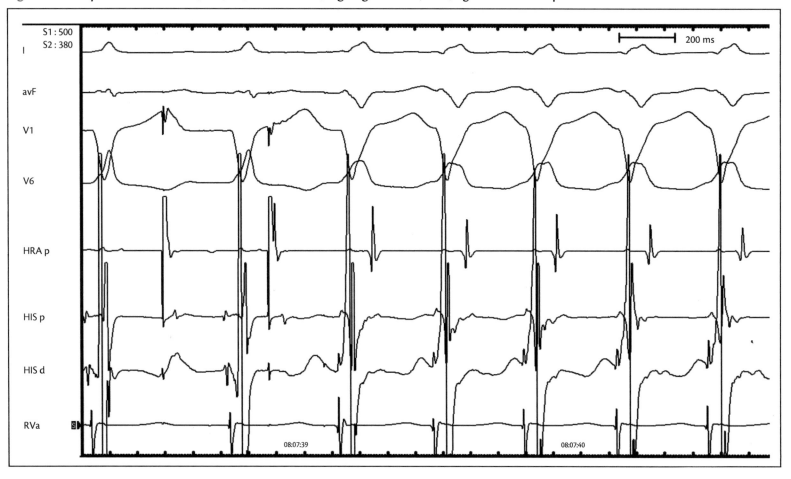

Question

The correct diagnosis is:

A   AVNRT

B   Atrial tachycardia

C   Orthodromic reciprocating tachycardia (ORT)

D   Ventricular tachycardia

E   Other

Answer

E   **Other**

Explanation

Differentiating wide complex tachycardia

During atrial pacing (the 1st beat), the His catheter has the activation sequence proximal to distal (antegrade His activation). During the 2nd paced beat, the His deflection (on proximal His) gets buried within the ventricle (block of the AV node, maximal pre-excitation) and antidromic tachycardia is induced. During tachycardia, the His activation sequence is reversed, and distal His is before proximal His. Therefore, the activation of the His bundle is retrograde during tachycardia, but still before ventricular activation. This is only possible in the presence of an extranodal pathway inserting in the fascicle just below the His bundle, most frequently the right bundle (Mahaim). Careful examination of the sequence of His bundle activation can lead to the correct diagnosis already at first glance in an otherwise highly complex diagnostic challenge.

The differential diagnosis of bundle branch re-entrant ventricular tachycardia (BBRVT) (number 4) is theoretically not fully excluded by this tracing. However, the induction with a relatively long AV interval (not so different from the basic interval seen at the first RR interval) makes it highly unlikely that only the right bundle is activated and the left bundle is completely blocked and able to conduct retrogradely for the re-entry circuit. Moreover, in BBRVT, the HV interval is not expected to be so short. The shortening of HV intervals during tachycardia and the reversal of His to proximal right bundle activation further argue against BBRVT where the HV interval would be equal to or longer than in sinus rhythm/atrial pacing.

Introduction to the case

Case 14 considers an 18-year-old male patient with paroxysmal palpitations. Adenosine injection (12mg bolus) was performed to evaluate the suspicion of pre-excitation on the ECG (Figure 14.1).

Figure 14.1 ECG—adenosine injection

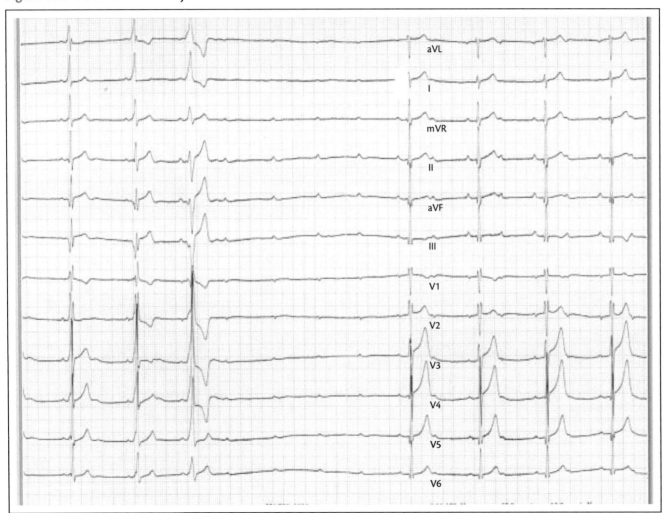

Question

This adenosine injection is associated with:

A An AV nodal block due to adenosine

B An accessory pathway conduction block due to adenosine

C Both

D None

Answer

C **Both**

Explanation

The wonderful effects of adenosine

The presence of an antegradely conducting extranodal accessory pathway was proven by demonstration of a pathway potential and successful ablation with loss of pre-excitation after 2s of radiofrequency delivery (Figure 14.2).

The initial beat shows an already slight pre-excitation. The QRS broadens in the 2nd and 3rd beats due to AV conduction slowing (with increased pre-excitation) and complete AV block (with full pre-excitation), respectively. Then total AV block ensues because also the accessory pathway is adenosine-sensitive and blocked. In the last four beats, AV nodal conduction resumes, but with persistent AP block; therefore, there is no pre-excitation during these final beats.

Figure 14.2 Presence of an antegradely conducting extranodal accessory pathway

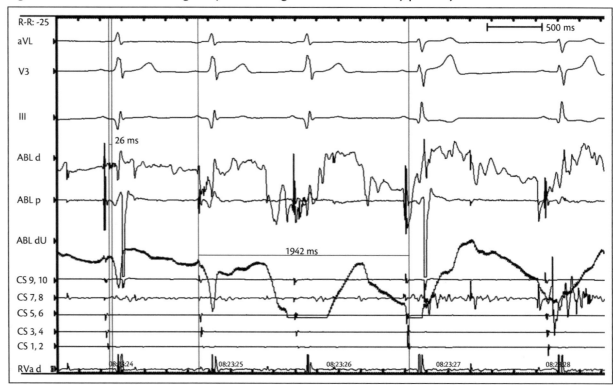

Introduction to the case

A woman, aged 35, with a long-standing history of paroxysmal SVT is admitted for an electrophysiological study (Figure 15.1). AVNRT with a cycle length of 450ms is easily induced (left panel). A concealed pathway is excluded by para-Hisian pacing and timed ventricular extrastimuli during tachycardia. Immediately after atrial burst pacing terminates the AVNRT, ventricular pacing at a para-Hisian position (i.e. from the distal pole of the His bundle catheter) is initiated at exactly the same cycle length as the tachycardia (right panel).

Figure 15.1 Comparison of timing and activation during AVNRT (left) and ventricular pacing at a para-Hisian site with the same cycle length as tachycardia. RAA: right atrial appendage; HBp till HBd: His bundle recordings from proximal to distal; PS: posteroseptal recording; CS: coronary sinus; A: atrial electrogram; H: His bundle deflection

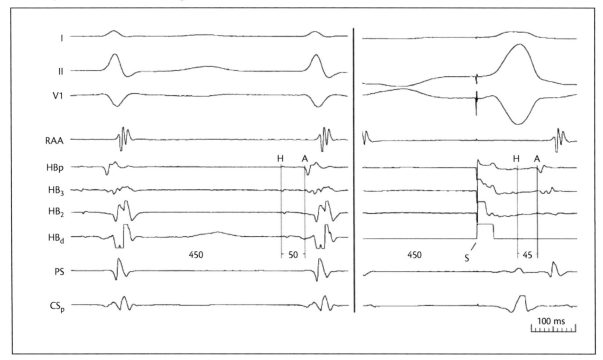

Question

When comparing the atrial activation sequence and HA interval during tachycardia and during ventricular pacing, the following conclusion can be made:

A There is evidence for a lower common pathway (LCP). The tachycardia is typical AVNRT

B There is no evidence for an LCP. The tachycardia is typical AVNRT

C There is evidence for an LCP. The tachycardia is atypical AVNRT

D There is no evidence for an LCP. The tachycardia is typical AVNRT

E It is circus movement tachycardia over a concealed accessory pathway after all

Answer

B There is no evidence for an LCP. The tachycardia is typical AVNRT

Explanation

Lower common pathway/1

The earliest atrial activation is present in the His bundle recording. That was not clear during tachycardia but became obvious during ventricular pacing, during which the atrial activation sequence was identical as that during tachycardia. The His-to-atrium (HA) interval during tachycardia, measured from the beginning of the most proximal antegrade His bundle potential (H) to the earliest atrial activation in the anterior septal area (A), was 50ms (HAt). During RV pacing at the same cycle length (right panel), the interval from the end of the most proximal retrograde His bundle potential (H) to the earliest atrial activation was 45ms (HAp). The difference (often labelled as ΔHA) was −5ms, which, together with the short HAp, excludes an LCP. This is a common finding in typical slow/ fast AVNRT but requires recording of the most proximal His bundle recording, which is only possible when pacing from a para-Hisian position.[1,2]

Compare also with Case 16.

References

1. Heidbüchel H, Jackman WM. Characterization of subforms of AV nodal reentrant tachycardia. *Europace* 2004; **6**: 316–29.

2. Miller JM, Rosenthal ME, Vassallo JA, Josephson ME. Atrioventricular nodal reentrant tachycardia: studies on upper and lower 'common pathways'. *Circulation* 1987; **75**: 930–40.

Introduction to the case

A woman with two recent admissions for sustained paroxysmal supraventricular tachycardia requiring intravenous conversion with adenosine is admitted for an electrophysiological study (Figure 16.1). AVNRT with a cycle length of 290ms is induced (left panel). A concealed pathway is excluded by para-Hisian pacing and timed ventricular extrastimuli during tachycardia. Immediately after atrial burst pacing terminates the AVNRT, ventricular pacing at a para-Hisian position (i.e. from the distal pole of the His bundle catheter) is initiated at exactly the same cycle length as the tachycardia (right panel). Pacing is performed with a low output (usually 2mA) to prevent direct capture of the His bundle. Therefore, retrograde His bundle activation can be discerned after the local ventricular electrogram during pacing.

Figure 16.1 Comparison of timing and activation during AVNRT (left) and ventricular pacing at a para-Hisian site with the same cycle length as tachycardia. RAA: right atrial appendage; HBp till HBd: His bundle recordings from proximal to distal; PS: posteroseptal recording; CS: coronary sinus; A: atrial electrogram; H: His bundle deflection

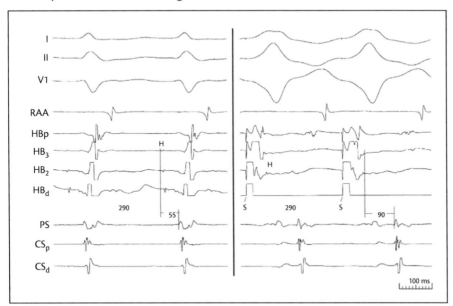

Question

When comparing the atrial activation sequence and HA interval during tachycardia and during ventricular pacing, the following conclusion can be made in this case:

A   There is evidence for an LCP. The tachycardia is typical AVNRT

B   There is no evidence for an LCP. The tachycardia is typical AVNRT

C   There is evidence for an LCP. The tachycardia is atypical AVNRT

D   There is no evidence for an LCP. The tachycardia is typical AVNRT

E   It is circus movement tachycardia over a concealed accessory pathway after all

Answer

C   There is evidence for an LCP. The tachycardia is atypical AVNRT

Explanation

Lower common pathway/2

The earliest retrograde atrial activation is present in the proximal CS recording, before the atrial activation in the His bundle recording. That was not clear during tachycardia but became obvious during ventricular pacing, during which the atrial activation sequence was identical as that during tachycardia. The HA interval during tachycardia, measured from the beginning of the most proximal antegrade His bundle potential (H) to the earliest atrial activation in the posterior septal area (A), was 55ms (HAt). During right ventricular pacing at the same cycle length (right panel), the interval from the end of the most proximal retrograde His bundle potential (H) to the earliest atrial activation was 90ms (HAp). The difference (often labelled as ΔHA) was 35ms. A ΔHA >15ms is indicative of an LCP in the nodal tissue between the turnaround point of the tachycardia and the His. The earliest atrial activation site and the long HAp indicate slow/slow AVNRT. Another sign for the presence of an LCP is Wenckebach VA conduction at a cycle length longer than, or equal to, the AVNRT cycle length (with 1:1 retrograde conduction).

The rationale for using the HA comparison technique is explained in Figures 16.2[1] and 16.3.[2] It requires recording of the most proximal His bundle recording, which is only possible when pacing from a para-Hisian position and an immediate transition from tachycardia to ventricular pacing to ensure a comparable autonomic tone during tachycardia and pacing. (Note: because of the need for recording the most proximal His bundle recording, ventricular pacing needs to be performed from a para-Hisian position. If pacing is performed from the right ventricular apex, there is a high likelihood that retrograde His bundle deflection and local ventricular electrogram will overlap, often leading to using a more distal right bundle potential as the 'His bundle'. This will lead to a false LCP, since in fact the proximal part of the right bundle will falsely be measured as the 'LCP').

An LCP is present in 84% of slow/slow AVNRT and in all patients with fast/slow AVNRT, but is absent in >90% of patients with typical slow/fast AVNRT.[2]

Compare also with Case 15.

Figure 16.2 The concept of ΔHA measurements.

Reproduced from J M Miller *et al*, Atrioventricular nodal reentrant tachycardia: studies on upper and lower 'common pathways'. *Circulation*, 1987 Vol. 75, No.5, with permission from Wolters Kluwer

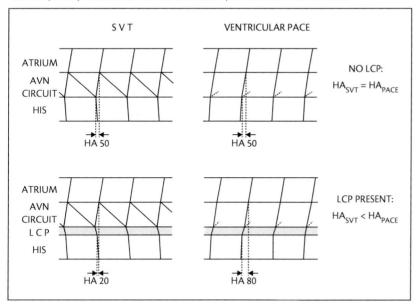

Figure 16.3 HA: His-to-atrium interval; rP: retrograde nodal conduction pathway (fast pathway or slow pathway); LCP: lower common pathway

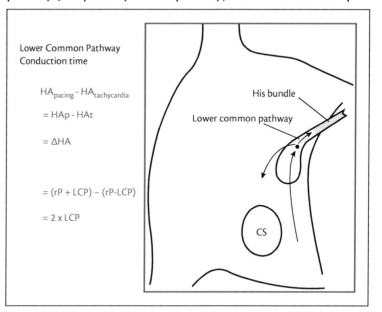

References

1. Miller JM, Rosenthal ME, Vassallo JA, Josephson ME. Atrioventricular nodal reentrant tachycardia: studies on upper and lower 'common pathways'. *Circulation* 1987; **75**: 930–40.

2. Heidbüchel H, Jackman WM. Characterization of subforms of AV nodal reentrant tachycardia. *Europace* 2004; **6**: 316–29.

Introduction to the case

This case discusses a 28-year-old woman with paroxysmal palpitations and spontaneous termination of clinical tachycardia with a non-conducted atrial beat (Figure 17.1).

Figure 17.1 Surface leads II and V1 and intracardiac recordings from the high right atrium (HRA), His bundle (HB), coronary sinus (CS), and right ventricular apex (RVA)

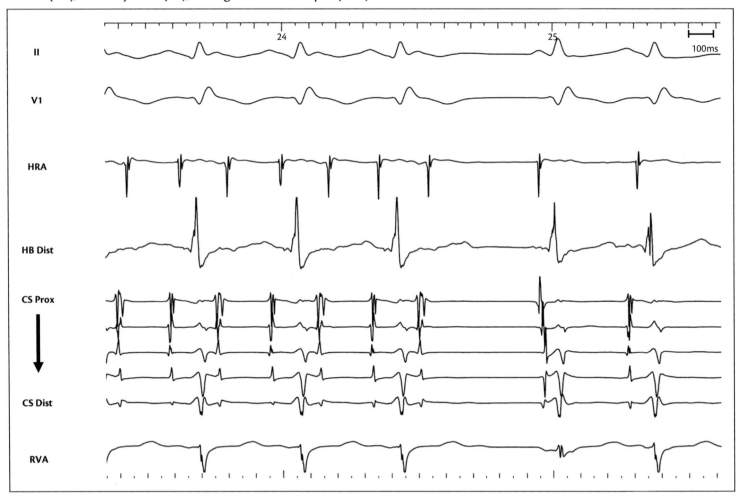

Question

In this tracing, termination of the wide complex QRS tachycardia with a non-conducted atrial beat:

A   Excludes AT as the mechanism

B   Suggests ventricular tachycardia (VT)

C   Could be compatible with AVNRT, orthodromic AVRT, as well as AT

D   Could be compatible with AT

E   Indicates infra-Hisian conduction block

Answer

D Could be compatible with AT

Explanation

Atrial tachycardia

This wide complex tachycardia is based upon an SVT with a right bundle block (A > V and 2:1 relation). Orthodromic AVRT is excluded because of the 2:1 A–V relation. Despite a rather simultaneous activation of the CS, the earliest A seems to be at the proximal CS. This SVT could be due to AVNRT with 2:1 conduction (in the presence of an LCP) or due to AT with 2:1 conduction.

Spontaneous termination of tachycardia with AV block occurs in 28% of tachycardias. It is a basic electrophysiology rule that, if tachycardia terminates with a non-conducted atrial beat, atrial tachycardia is excluded (because fortuitous occurrence of both termination of AT and AV block is highly unlikely). However, this basic rule only applies to SVT with 1:1 A–V conduction. During AT with spontaneous 2:1 AV block, the likelihood of termination by a non-conducted atrial beat is 50%, and therefore spontaneous termination of tachycardia with AV block does not exclude AT. In this patient, an ectopic AT was successfully ablated (right superior pulmonary vein (RSPV)).

Introduction to the case

A bipolar recording is often preferred in the catheterization laboratory because it reduces both 50/60Hz interference and remote activation, compared to a unipolar recording. The bipolar recording also has, however, several disadvantages. The interpretation of the configuration of a bipolar electrogram (Figure 18.1) is not as straightforward as that of a unipolar one, and the signal is direction-dependent. This hampers detection of the activation time in the bipolar electrogram.

Figure 18.1 Activation time in the bipolar electrogram

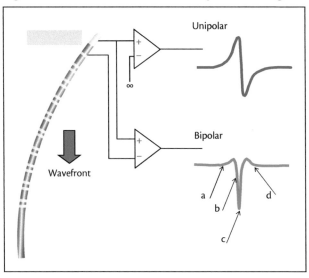

Question

Where is the activation time in the bipolar electrogram shown in the figure (green tracing)?

A   At the beginning of the electrogram

B   At the point of the steepest negative dV/dt

C   At the time of the peak negative value

D   At the end of the signal

Answer

C At the time of the peak negative value

Explanation

Bipolar electrogram morphology

If the poles of a bipolar electrode are close together, a bipolar electrogram is virtually the first derivative (dV/dt) of the unipolar electrogram.[1] The simultaneous recording of intracellular and extracellular electrograms from the same site has shown that the point of the fastest upstroke of the action potential (which marks the depolarization of the myocardial cell) corresponds with the point of the steepest negative downstroke in the unipolar extracellular electrogram.[2] The latter corresponds with the largest negative value in the bipolar electrogram. One should realize that if the wavefront comes from the opposite direction, the unipolar electrogram remains virtually the same, whereas the bipolar signal inverts and the activation time corresponds with the peak positive value.

References

1. de Bakker JMT, Hauer RNW, Simmers TA (1995). Activation mapping: unipolar versus bipolar recording. In: DP Zipes, J Jalife (eds.). *Cardiac Electrophysiology: From Cell to Bedside*, 2nd edn. Philadelphia: WB Saunders Company, pp. 1068–78.

2. Janse MJ (1986). Electrophysiology and electrocardiology of acute myocardial ischemia. *Can J Cardiol* **Suppl A**: 46A–52A.

CASE 18

72

Introduction to the case

Differential pacing manoeuvres were performed to evaluate bidirectional cavo-tricuspid isthmus conduction block for typical flutter ablation. The catheters were positioned as shown in Figure 19.1.

Figure 19.1 Differential pacing manoeuvre to evaluate bidirectional cavo-tricuspid isthmus conduction block. The ablation catheter was placed medially from the line and pulled back slightly to record the electrograms in the upper panel (a-c) and pushed further towards the ventricle to record the electrograms in the lower panel (e-g). ABL D: distal ablation; ABL P: proximal ablation; LRA D: distal low right atrium; LRA P: proximal low right atrium; Ω: pacing channel

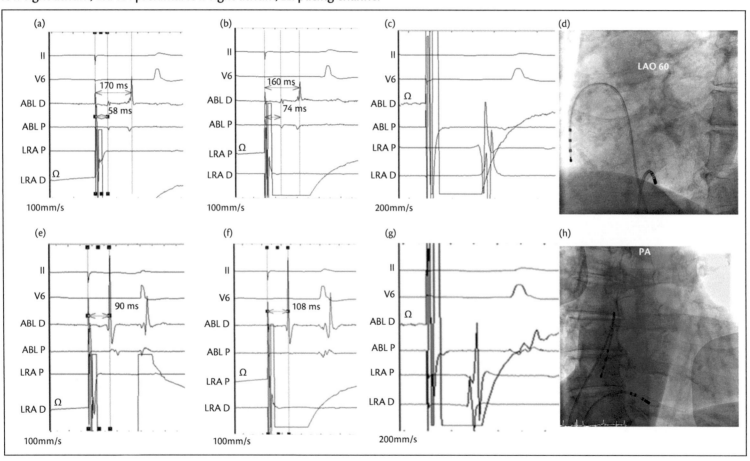

Question

What do you observe?

A   Unidirectional block shown on the caval aspect of the isthmus

B   Unidirectional block shown on the ventricular aspect of the isthmus

C   Bidirectional block shown on the ventricular aspect of the isthmus

D   Bidirectional conduction shown on the ventricular aspect of the isthmus

E   Bidirectional block shown on the caval and ventricular aspects of the isthmus

Answer

D   Bidirectional conduction shown on the ventricular aspect of the isthmus

Explanation

Evaluation of bidirectional cavo-tricuspid isthmus block by differential pacing manoeuvres

The differential pacing manoeuvre at the caval aspect of the isthmus suggests bidirectional block (in the top panels, note the far-field double potential on ABL P and ABL D). However, differential pacing manoeuvres from the ventricular aspect of the isthmus show residual conduction (in the bottom panels, the stimulus to atrial potential interval on ABL is shorter when pacing from LRA D, compared to LRA P, with a distal to proximal sequence on the LRA catheter when pacing from ABL D medially to the line of ablation). This example shows the importance of mapping the entire ablation line to confirm bidirectional block. When performing differential pacing, the LRA catheter should be positioned close to the ablation line, ideally with a stimulus to first potential duration of <50ms, otherwise residual conduction may be missed.[1,2] It was not possible in this case to position the non-steerable quadripolar diagnostic catheter in a stable position closer to the line of ablation (the stimulus to first potential interval was 58ms). Additional radiofrequency applications were performed on the ventricular aspect of the line, resulting in bidirectional block (Figure 19.2).

References

1. Shah DC, Takahashi A, Jaïs P, Hocini M, Clémenty J, Haïssaguerre M. Local electrogram-based criteria of cavotricuspid isthmus block. *J Cardiovasc Electrophysiol* 1999; **10**: 662–9.

2. Shah D, Haïssaguerre M, Takahashi A, Jaïs P, Hocini M, Clémenty J. Differential pacing for distinguishing block from persistent conduction through an ablation line. *Circulation* 2000; **102**: 1517–22.

Figure 19.2 Differential pacing manoeuvre showing bidirectional block of the cavo-tricuspid isthmus. ABL D: distal ablation; ABL P: proximal ablation; LRA D: distal low right atrium; LRA P: proximal low right atrium; Ω: pacing channel

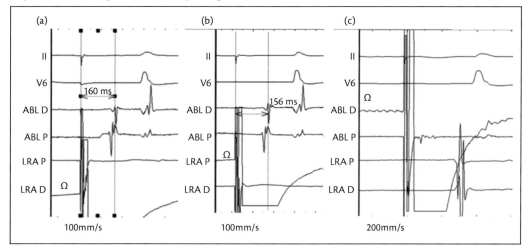

Introduction to the case

This case describes a 53-year-old woman and the evaluation of isolation of the RSPV at the end of encircling the right veins (pacing during ongoing atrial fibrillation) (Figure 20.1).

Figure 20.1 (a) RSPV after encircling (during atrial fibrillation). (b) Slow pacing (S1S1 600ms) from within the encircled pulmonary veins (PVs). Surface leads II and V2, and intracardiac recordings from the coronary sinus (CS), Lasso catheter at the LA–PV junction of the RSPV, and the ablation catheter positioned within the circle (ABLC)

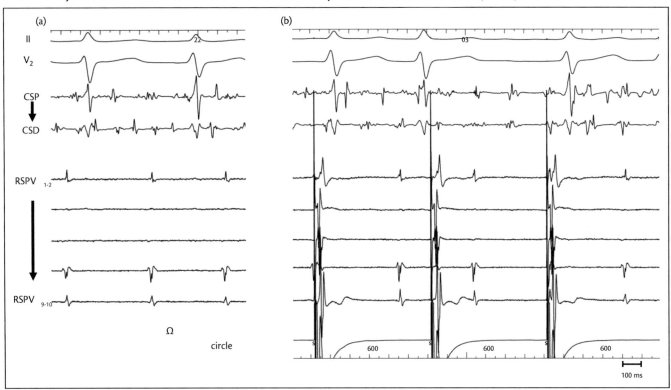

Question

The tracings show:

A   The RSPV is not isolated (no entry block)

B   The RSPV is characterized by exit block

C   The RSPV is isolated (entry block during atrial fibrillation)

D   The diagnosis of entry block cannot be verified during atrial fibrillation

E   The RSPV reveals bigeminy

Answer

C **The RSPV is isolated (entry block during atrial fibrillation)**

Explanation

Entry block during atrial fibrillation

Figure 20.1a: the Lasso was positioned at the RSPV after encircling the right veins during atrial fibrillation. The residual atrial potentials are either PV potentials or far-field potentials. The longer cycle length (compared to the atrial fibrillation cycle length) suggests an ablation-induced LA–PV delay (no entry block).

Figure 20.1b: slow pacing (S1S1 600ms) from within the circle is characterized by pacing spikes instantaneously followed by local high-frequency potentials on the Lasso catheter (capture of PV sleeves). Capture of PV sleeves during atrial fibrillation can only be obtained if the encircled area is completely isolated (entry block). This indicates that the residual atrial potentials are far-field recordings (in this case proven to originate from the superior vena cava (SVC)). Isolation of the encircled area (downstream electrical silence beyond the line of block) can also be appreciated by the absence of any recording of local atrial potentials on the ablation catheter (even beyond the saturation window).

Note: variable degrees of entry block from the right atrium to the SVC are a consistent finding during atrial fibrillation.

Introduction to the case

Case 21 discusses a 34-year-old man with recurrent palpitations (Figure 21.1).

Figure 21.1 Intravenous administration of adenosine bolus. Surface leads I, III, aVL, and V1, and intracardiac recording from His

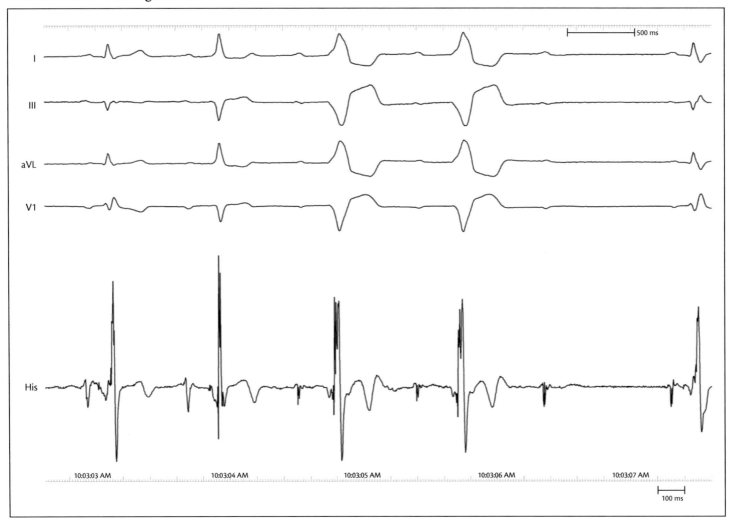

Question

This tracing is compatible with:

A   Atrio-fascicular pathway

B   Progressive aberrancy over the left bundle

C   Nodo-fascicular pathway

D   Right-sided PVCs

E   None of the above answers

Answer

A Atrio-fascicular pathway

Explanation

Mahaim

Mahaim fibre physiology during administration of adenosine. In sinus rhythm, there is typically little or no pre-excitation (1st sinus beat is characterized by right bundle branch block morphology, and normal AH and HV intervals).

The 2nd beat is characterized by adenosine-induced prolongation of the AH and A-delta interval with signs of pre-excitation and shortening of the HV interval.

The 3rd and 4th beats are maximally pre-excited (most likely nodal block), while the isoelectric A-delta and AH intervals further prolong.

The His deflection gets buried within the V deflection (conform with retrograde His bundle activation). The onset of QRS precedes HB activation.

The 5th beat is characterized by block at the atrio-fascicular pathway (and node).

Introduction to the case

Case 22 discusses a 48-year-old woman with persistent AT. The patient underwent prior mitral valve annulovalvuloplasty (rheumatic stenosis), surgical exclusion of the left atrial appendage, and intraoperative isolation of the PVs and posterior wall ('box lesion'). During an electrophysiological study, atrial pacing was performed from the proximal CS (Figure 22.1a), distal CS (Figure 22.1b), and left atrial anterior wall (Figure 22.1c).

Figure 22.1 (a) Surface leads I, II, V1, and V6, and intracardiac recordings from the distal to proximal bipoles of the coronary sinus (Dec 1-2: distal CS; Dec 9-10: proximal CS). (b) Idem as (a). (c) Surface lead V1 and intracardiac recordings from the distal to proximal bipoles of the coronary sinus (Dec 1-2: distal CS; Dec 7-8: proximal CS). Intracardiac recordings from distal and proximal bipoles of the ablation catheter (ABL); paper speed: 100mm/s

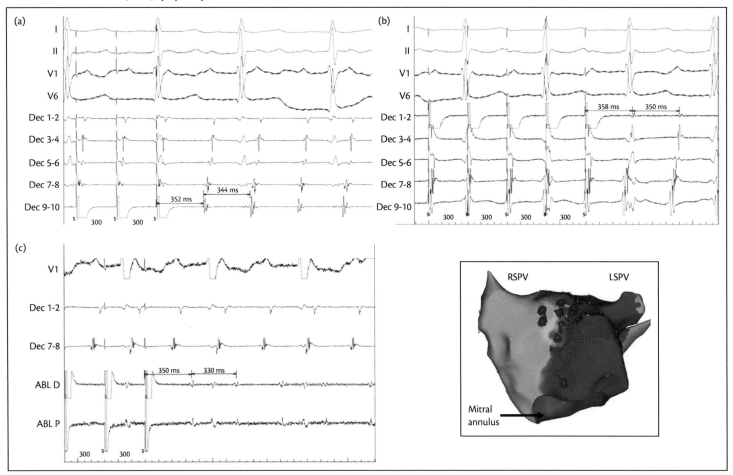

Question

The following is true:

A   Entrainment pacing is consistent with left septal re-entry

B   Entrainment pacing is compatible with right-sided flutter

C   Posterior left atrial wall entrainment should be assessed to define diagnosis

D   The anterior wall or mitral isthmus should be considered for ablation

E   Entrainment mapping is consistent with clockwise perimitral atrial flutter

Answer

D   **The anterior wall or mitral isthmus should be considered for ablation**

Explanation

Entrainment pacing to differentiate intra-atrial re-entrant tachycardia/1

Entrainment mapping shows a post-pacing interval (PPI)-TCL within 30ms at all pacing sites, indicating that perimitral atrial flutter is the diagnosis, without the need for further pacing manoeuvres.

CS recordings indicate a counterclockwise perimitral activation.

Typically, the ablation target for perimitral flutter is the mitral isthmus. This, however, can be difficult to achieve, warranting epicardial ablation via the CS in up to 30% of cases.

In this case, the anterior wall can be considered for ablation as well. The local recording (Figure 22.1c) is consistent with the critical isthmus (note the mesodiastolic potential on the mapping tracing) that was found to be a quite narrow site of slow conduction between the anterior mitral annulus and the scarred area caused by the roof line (as part of the box lesion) and left atrial appendage suture.

A few radiofrequency pulses at this site allowed tachycardia termination with persistent non-inducibility.

This case underlines how matching electrophysiological findings with the clinical context is of paramount importance to choose the best ablation strategy (the maximum result with the lowest radiofrequency application).

Introduction to the case

A 10-pole circular mapping catheter (Figure 23.1) is positioned in the RSPV after PV isolation and proven entrance block. Pacing at decremental pacing outputs via the circular mapping catheter is shown.

Figure 23.1 A: bipolar electrograms from the 10-pole ablation catheter; CS: coronary sinus catheter

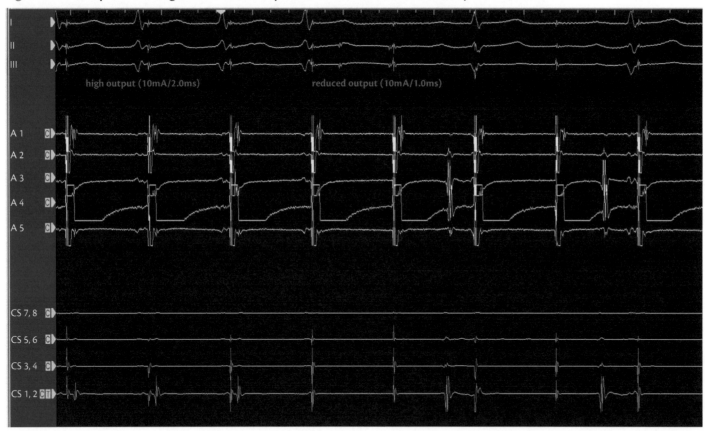

Question

What happens during pacing with high output (A) and then with reduced output (B)?

A   (A) local capture with conduction to the left atrium (exit conduction) and (B) loss of capture

B   (A) far-field capture and (B) local capture with exit conduction

C   (A) far-field capture and (B) local capture with exit block

D   (A) local capture with exit block and (B) far-field capture with exit block

E   (A) local capture with exit block and (B) far-field capture with exit conduction

Answer

C (A) far-field capture and (B) local capture with exit block

Explanation

Pulmonary vein capture with exit block and intermittent far-field atrial capture

(A) The first part indicates far-field capture during high-output PV pacing, capturing not only local tissue, but also far-field left atrial tissue with 1:1 activation and short conduction time to the CS electrograms.

(B) Lowering pacing output indicates local capture of near-field PV–myocardial sleeves with exit block to the left atrium. During sinus rhythm, the electrodes facing the posterior wall (A3, A4) reveal far-field electrograms from the adjacent posterior left atrium. This case illustrates that proof of exit block can be hidden by far-field capture.

Introduction to the case

Dispersion of the action potential duration (APD) is considered to be a parameter for arrhythmogenicity. Detection of the action potential requires intracellular recordings, which are not feasible in the clinical setting. As a substitute for the APD, the activation recovery interval (ARI) is used (Figure 24.1), which can be derived from unipolar recordings as the interval from the depolarization to the repolarization. Although the depolarization can be determined easily in a unipolar recording, the point of repolarization is less clear.

Figure 24.1 Activation recovery interval (ARI)

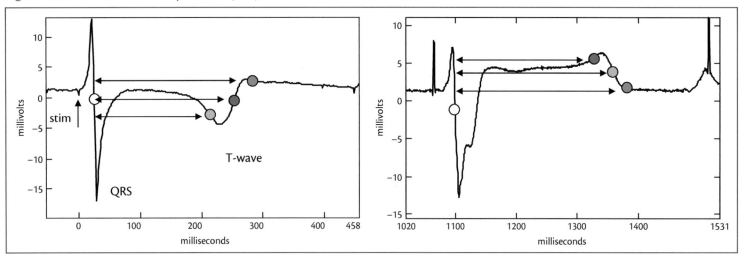

Question

Which interval in the electrograms marks the ARI?

A   The interval from the white to the green dot

B   The interval from the white to the red dot

C   The interval from the white to the blue dot

D   The interval from the white to the red dot for the left tracing and the interval from the white to the green dot for the right tracing.

Answer

B   The interval from the white to the red dot

Explanation

Activation recovery interval

In a unipolar electrogram, the activation time is the point of the steepest negative deflection in the depolarizing phase of the signal (the white dot in the signals). Simultaneous intra- and extracellular recordings have shown that the repolarization corresponds to the point of the steepest positive deflection in the repolarizing phase of the unipolar electrogram.[1] It does not matter whether the configuration of the repolarization wave is only positive (right tracing), negative (left tracing), or biphasic; the time of repolarization always corresponds with the point of the steepest upstroke.[2,3] In this case, the repolarization (T-wave) is flat, and the point of repolarization cannot be determined.

References

1. Coronel R, de Bakker JM, Wilms-Schopman FJ, *et al.* Monophasic action potentials and activation recovery intervals as measures of ventricular action potential duration: experimental evidence to resolve some controversies. *Heart Rhythm* 2006; **3**: 1043–50.

2. Gepstein L, Hayam G, Ben Haim SA. Activation-repolarization coupling in the normal swine myocardium. *Circulation* 1997; **96**: 4036–43.

3. Haws CW, Lux RL. Correlation between *in vivo* transmembrane action potential duration and activation-recovery intervals from electrograms. Effects of interventions that alter repolarization time. *Circulation* 1990; **81**: 281–8.

Introduction to the case

A 69-year-old patient with palpitations had the following recording during an electro-physiological study (Figure 25.1). The sustained narrow complex tachycardia was initiated spontaneously.

Figure 25.1 Electrophysiological study

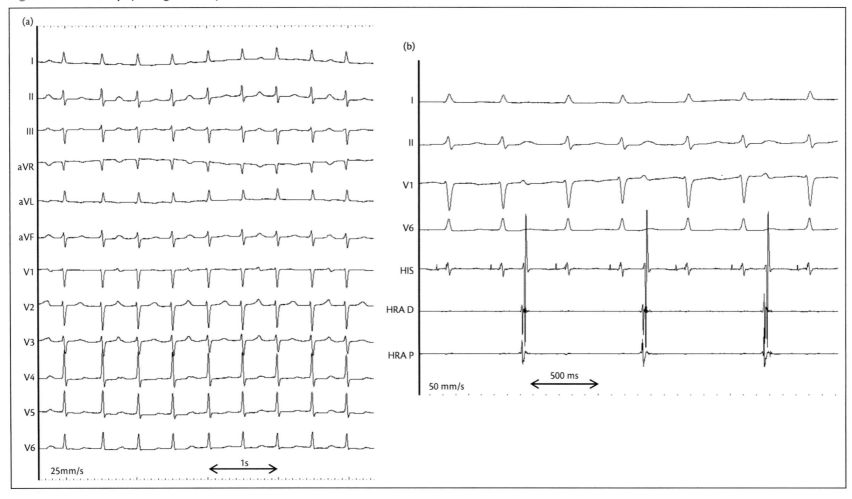

Question

What is the most likely diagnosis?

A   AT

B   AVNRT with 2:1 retrograde block

C   Automatic junctional tachycardia with 2:1 retrograde block

D   Junctional bigeminy

E   Non-re-entrant atrioventricular nodal tachycardia

Answer

E   **Non-re-entrant atrioventricular nodal tachycardia**

Explanation

Double fire tachycardia

The tracing shows a narrow complex tachycardia with a 1:2 A:V ratio (ruling out AT). AVNRT or junctional tachycardia with a 2:1 retrograde block (which is extremely rare) are incompatible with the P-wave morphology (which are positive in the inferior leads), as well as the repetitive 'long–short' H–H intervals. Junctional bigeminy is unlikely, given the sustained nature of the tachycardia and the absence of any retrograde P-waves. Non-re-entrant atrioventricular nodal tachycardia (otherwise known as 'double fire tachycardia') is due to dual AV nodal conduction, with anterograde conduction via both a fast and a slow pathway (the AH intervals are shown in Figure 25.2), resulting in 'double fire' of each P-wave.[1,2] The finding often coexists with AVNRT and is treated in the same manner by radiofrequency modification of the slow pathway.

References

1. Burri H, Hoffmann J, Zimmermann M. Double fire tachycardia. *Heart* 2012; **98**: 958.

2. Zimmermann M, Testuz A, Schmutz M, *et al.* Narrow-complex tachycardia with cycle length alternans: what is the mechanism? *Heart Rhythm* 2009; **6**: 1238–9.

Figure 25.2   AH intervals

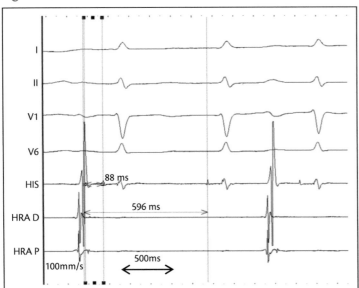

Introduction to the case

A 36-year-old woman had an electrophysiological study performed for palpitations. Atrial pacing with one premature beat triggered a narrow complex tachycardia, which was interrupted by an intrinsic ventricular premature beat (Figure 26.1).

Figure 26.1 Interruption of tachycardia by a ventricular premature beat. His d: distal His; His p: proximal His; LRA d: distal low right atrium; LRA p: proximal low right atrium; RV: right ventricle

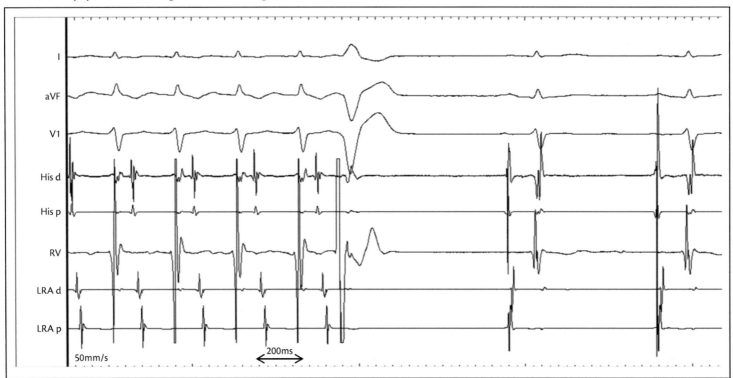

Question

Which of the following statements is true?

A   AT can be excluded

B   AVNRT can be excluded

C   AVRT can be excluded

D   Answers A and C are correct

E   None of the above are correct

Answer

A AT can be excluded

Explanation

Interruption of a supraventricular tachycardia by a ventricular premature beat

A regular SVT with an RP < PR interval can be observed, with a caudo-cranial atrial activation sequence. The septal VA interval is >70ms, with a differential diagnosis comprising AT, AVNRT, and AVRT. However, the ventricular premature beat (which is probably mechanical from the RV catheter as electrical activity in this channel is early and the surface ECG is compatible with an RV apical origin) interrupts the arrhythmia *without activating the atrium*. This rules out AT, which may only be interrupted by a ventricular premature beat if there is retrograde conduction. AVNRT may only be excluded if the ventricular premature beat occurs during the His refractory period (which would result in an entrance block into the AV node). The His potential is, however, not clearly seen on the catheter, but the premature beat is probably early enough and close enough to the conduction tissue to conduct retrogradely into the AV node, thus interrupting the tachycardia. AVRT would have been excluded if the VA interval during tachycardia (measured from the onset of the QRS to the earliest A) had been <70ms,[1,2] which is not the case here. The tachycardia in this instance may be interrupted by the same mechanism as for AVNRT, or otherwise by a retrograde block of the accessory pathway.

References

1. Benditt DG, Pritchett EL, Smith WM, Gallagher JJ. Ventriculoatrial intervals: diagnostic use in paroxysmal supraventricular tachycardia. *Ann Intern Med* 1979; **91**: 161–6.

2. Knight BP, Ebinger M, Oral H, *et al*. Diagnostic value of tachycardia features and pacing maneuvers during paroxysmal supraventricular tachycardia. *J Am Coll Cardiol* 2000; **36**: 574–82.

Introduction to the case

This case shows an example of a 23-year-old man with short palpitations at rest (Figure 27.1).

Figure 27.1 Short palpitations at rest

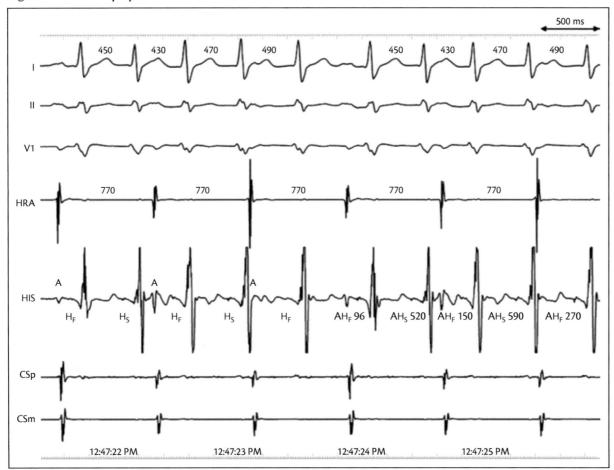

Question

The mechanism of tachycardia is:

A   VT

B   AVNRT with an upper common pathway

C   Sinus rhythm with an intermittent dual ventricular response

D   Atrial fibrillation

E   Junctional tachycardia

Answer

C **Sinus rhythm with an intermittent dual ventricular response**

Explanation

Sinus rhythm with dual nodal response

The presence of (1) more QRS complexes than regular P-waves and (2) group beating with regular irregularity suggests the presence of a dual ventricular response with Wenckebach behaviour during normal sinus rhythm. The intracardiac high right atrium recording indeed shows regular AA intervals. The 1st P-wave initiates a double His response due to conduction over a fast pathway (AHf = 96ms) and a slow pathway (Ahs = 520ms). The 2nd P-wave also conducts over the fast and slow pathways with an AH interval of, respectively, 150ms and 590ms, suggesting Wenckebach behaviour in these pathways. The 3rd P-wave blocks in the slow pathway and only conducts over the fast pathway with an AHf of 270ms. The 4th P-wave conducts again over both pathways, but surprisingly the AHf is again 96ms. This suggests that the progressive increase of the AHf interval within a group is dependent upon conduction over the slow pathway in the previous beat and is not due to Wenckebach behaviour in the fast pathway per se. A possible explanation could be the presence of an LCP with decremental conduction properties. A block in the slow pathway prevents activation of the LCP, facilitating conduction of the next impulse coming over the fast pathway.

Introduction to the case

This case is about a 45-year-old woman with palpitations and documented narrow complex tachycardia. The following observations are made at an electrophysiological study after a narrow QRS tachycardia with a cycle length of 400ms had been induced. Ventricular overdrive pacing is performed at 30ms faster than the TCL. The tracing (Figure 28.1) shows the termination of overdrive pacing.

Figure 28.1 Surface leads II, aVF, V1, and V6, and intracardiac recordings from the high right atrium (HRA), the proximal, mid, and distal bipoles of the His bundle (His), the proximal to distal bipoles of the coronary sinus (CS), and the right ventricular apex (RVA)

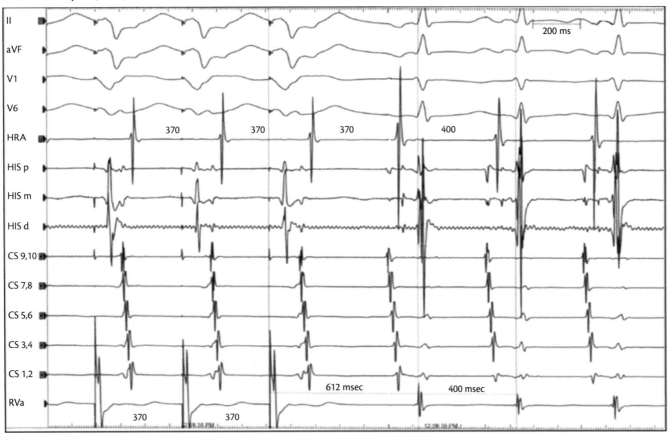

Question

The tracing proves:

A   The tachycardia is atypical (fast/slow) AVNRT

B   The tachycardia is AVRT

C   The tachycardia is AT

D   Failure of atrial entrainment with ventricular overdrive pacing

E   The tachycardia is typical (slow/fast) AVNRT

Answer

A The tachycardia is atypical (fast/slow) AVNRT

Explanation

Ventricular overdrive pacing during supraventricular tachycardia/2

The tracing demonstrates ventricular overdrive pacing at 30ms faster than the TCL, with acceleration of the atrium to the same rate. On termination of pacing, there is an apparent VAAV response. However, on closer inspection of the AA timing post-pacing, it is evident that the 2nd atrial beat after the last stimulated beat is still following the pacing cycle length (370ms). This is a pseudo-VAAV response as the atrium had been captured by either the slow pathway or a slowly conducting bypass tract retrogradely to match the ventricular pacing rate. The pseudo-VAAV response is typically seen with long RP tachycardias. Given that this is in essence a VAV response, the differential diagnosis lies between AVNRT or AVRT (over an accessory pathway with a long conduction time). The tachycardia has a short AH interval and a long VA interval, with the earliest atrial activation at the proximal CS. AVRT would constitute participation of the ventricles to the tachycardia circuit. Since the retrograde activation sequence is earliest septally, the PPI and stimulus-to-A intervals can be employed to differentiate between the two, even with pacing from the RV apex, as in this case—a PPI-TCL of >115ms with apical pacing is consistent with AVNRT, as in this case (PPI = 212ms).[1] Alternatively, one could introduce ventricular extrastimuli from the posterobasal RV at the time of His refractoriness or entrainment from that site, which would differentiate even more clearly. The slow pathway was successfully ablated in this patient with an atypical fast/slow AVNRT.

References

1. Michaud GF, Tada H, Chough S, *et al.* Differentiation of atypical atrioventricular node re-entrant tachycardia from orthodromic reciprocating tachycardia using a septal accessory pathway by the response to ventricular pacing. *J Am Coll Cardiol* 2001; **38**: 1163–7.

Introduction to the case

A woman, aged 41, with AVNRT is discussed in this case. Twenty seconds after starting ablation of the slow pathway (over the posteroseptal area, between the tricuspid annulus and the ostium of the CS) and immediately inducing junctional rhythm, suddenly the following tracing (Figure 29.1) is recorded.

Figure 29.1 Intracardiac recordings 20s after the start of ablation of the slow pathway in a patient with AVNRT. RAA: right atrial appendage; HBp till HBd: His bundle recordings from proximal to distal; PS: posteroseptal position (between tricuspid annulus and coronary sinus ostium); CS: coronary sinus; rA: retrograde atrial activation; SR: sinus rhythm

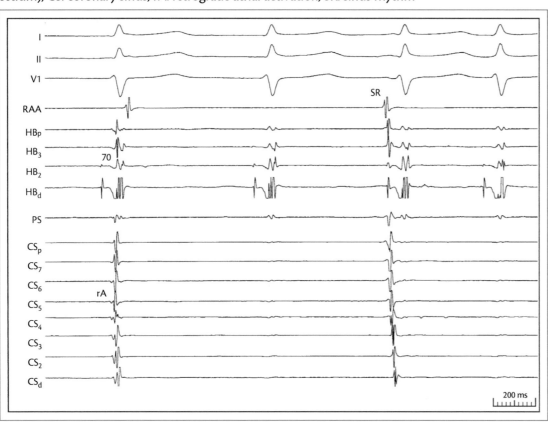

Question

Which action cannot be recommended?

A   Immediate termination of energy delivery

B   Immediate termination. Only when (a) absence of ablation endpoint (non-inducibility and/or absence of 1:1 antegrade conduction over the slow pathway), (b) certainty that the AVNRT subform is *slow/slow*, and (c) the energy is delivered not higher than the upper margin of the CS ostium—consider continuation

C   Immediate termination. Only when (a) absence of ablation endpoint (non-inducibility and/or absence of 1:1 antegrade conduction over the slow pathway), (b) certainty that the AVNRT subform is *fast/slow*, and (c) the energy is delivered not higher than the upper margin of the CS ostium—consider continuation

D   Immediate termination. Only when (a) absence of ablation endpoint (non-inducibility and/or absence of 1:1 antegrade conduction over the slow pathway), (b) certainty that the AVNRT subform is *slow/fast*, and (c) the energy is delivered not higher than the upper margin of the CS ostium—consider continuation

E   Continuation after starting atrial pacing at a slightly faster rate

Answer

D **Immediate termination. Only when (a) absence of ablation endpoint (non-inducibility and/or absence of 1:1 antegrade conduction over the slow pathway), (b) certainty that the AVNRT subform is *slow/fast*, and (c) the energy is delivered not higher than the upper margin of the CS ostium—consider continuation**

Explanation

Slow pathway ablation

Induction of junctional rhythm during ablation of the slow AV nodal pathway, as is occurring in this tracing, indicates heating of the approaches of the AV node and is often a sign (albeit not very specific) for effective slow pathway ablation. This automaticity usually conducts both towards the ventricles and the atrium. In the tracing, the junctional beats are suddenly not conducted to the atrium anymore. This indicates that the retrograde conduction path is compromised. Since most AVNRT forms are typical slow/fast, the retrograde conduction path usually is the fast (physiologic) pathway. Hence, non-conduction signals imminent damage to the fast pathway which could result in AV block. Therefore, immediate cessation of energy delivery is mandatory if the AV subform is typical slow/fast and continued radiofrequency delivery is highly contraindicated.

However, if prior evaluation of the AVNRT subform (before the 1st ablation attempt!) indicated an atypical form (fast/slow or slow/slow), junctional rhythm with retrograde block can be anticipated during ablation, since the junctional rhythm has to use the same pathway that is being ablated for retrograde conduction to the atrium. In such circumstances, a block towards the atrium may even be required for effective ablation of the arrhythmia circuit.

Nevertheless, one should assure that energy delivery is not higher than the upper margin of the CS ostium and that there was no retrograde fast pathway conduction during ventricular pacing at the same cycle length as the junctional rhythm before the ablation. This calls for good AVNRT subform differentiation before the start of radiofrequency delivery!

Finally, after interruption of the initial radiofrequency delivery, it is recommended to be prepared during the next radiofrequency application to immediately start atrial pacing at a slightly faster rate than the junctional rhythm, as is shown in Figure 29.2, in which the last two beats show AV conduction over the fast pathway. This enables online evaluation of the integrity of antegrade AV nodal conduction and safe continuation of the ablation to reach the desired endpoint.

Figure 29.2 Radiofrequency application and atrial pacing at a slightly faster rate than the junctional rhythm

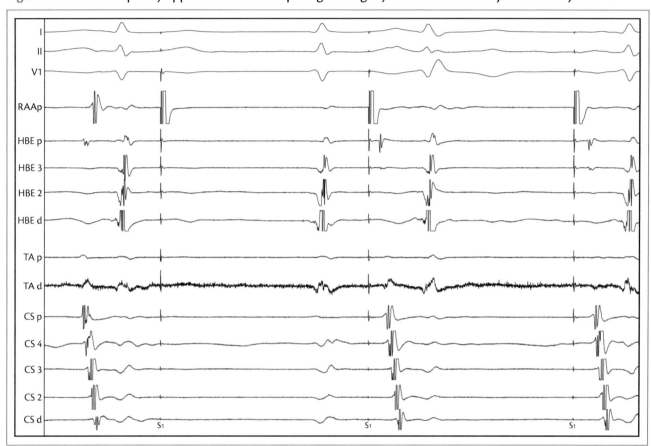

Introduction to the case

This case discusses a 42-year-old schoolteacher. The patient underwent slow pathway ablation for AVNRT and during post-ablation testing developed this tachycardia. A His-refractory premature atrial complex (PAC) was delivered during the tachycardia (Figure 30.1). What is the most likely mechanism of the tachycardia and would you continue ablation of the slow pathway?

Figure 30.1 His-refractory PAC delivered during tachycardia

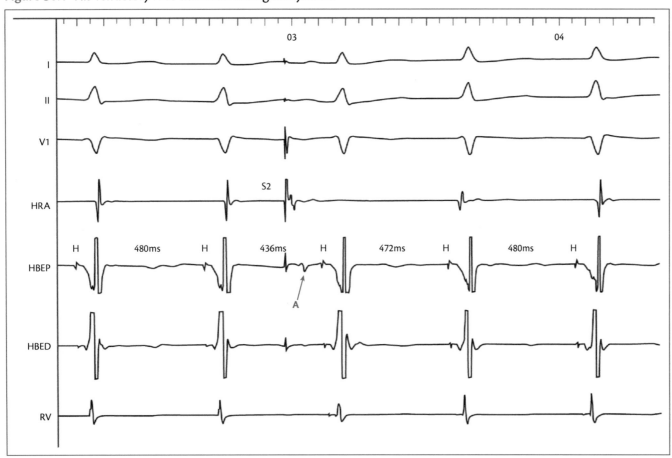

Question

The tracing proves:

A   AVNRT

B   AVRT

C   Junctional tachycardia

D   Nodo-fascicular AVNRT

Answer

C Junctional tachycardia

Explanation

Is the slow pathway ablated, or isn't it?

The PAC (S2) advances the immediate His by 44ms, and the tachycardia continues. The red arrow indicates the local atrial activation on the His recording catheter that occurs before the His bundle activation. This advancement of the immediate His by a PAC with continuation of tachycardia indicates junctional tachycardia as the mechanism, and further ablations are not necessary.[1] This is because the advancement of the His requires fast pathway activation. If the tachycardia was AVNRT, then it would be terminated by the PAC as the fast pathway would still be refractory. The tachycardia cannot be an AVRT, as the VA time is too short during tachycardia (simultaneous activation of V and A <60ms on the His), and an atrio-fascicular tachycardia would have evidence of pre-excitation both during tachycardia and particularly post-PAC.

References

1. Padanilam BJ, Manfredi JA, Steinberg LA, Olson JA, Fogel RI, Prystowsky EN. Differentiating junctional tachycardia and atrioventricular node re-entry tachycardia based on response to atrial extrastimulus pacing. *J Am Coll Cardiol* 2008; **52**: 1711–17.

Introduction to the case

An 8-year-old girl with recurrent palpitations is discussed in Case 31. There is no overt cardiomyopathy or evident P-wave enlargement. During an electrophysiological study, the following tracings are recorded at induction (Figure 31.1a) and termination (Figure 31.1b) of the clinical tachycardia. Catheters are placed as shown in the left anterior oblique (LAO) fluoroscopic image (Figure 31.1c).

Figure 31.1 Surface leads I and III, and intracardiac recordings from the distal to proximal bipoles of the coronary sinus. DCS 1: distal CS; MCS 2–4: middle CS; PCS 5: proximal CS; HBE: distal and proximal His; ABL: distal and proximal bipoles of the ablation catheter

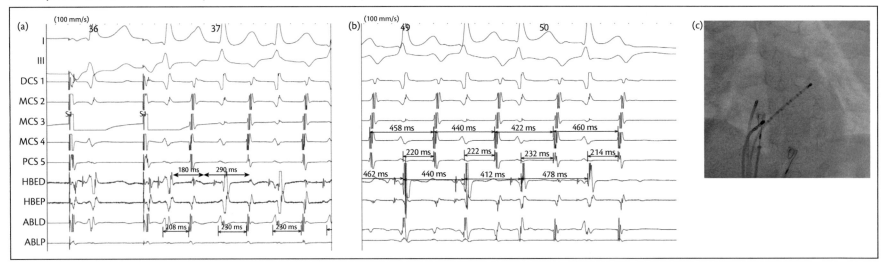

Question

Which is the most likely diagnosis?

A   Fast/slow AVNRT

B   PJRT (orthodromic AVRT associated with a concealed slow posteroseptal accessory pathway)

C   AT

D   Dual nodal response

E   None of the above

Answer

B   PJRT (orthodromic AVRT associated with a concealed slow posteroseptal accessory pathway)

Explanation

Differentiating narrow QRS tachycardia

The tracing shows induction and termination of a long R–P tachycardia, with inferoseptal earliest atrial activation, near the CS os (ABLd); this can be caused by fast/slow AVNRT, slow/slow AVNRT, PJRT, and AT.[1-3] However, a differential diagnosis in this case can be obtained with the subsequent observations:

- AT is ruled out because tachycardia terminates with atrial activation; furthermore, just before termination, cycle length variation is evident, with V–V variations that precede coherent A–A variations.
- Differentiating atypical AVNRT from PJRT might be more challenging. In both cases, a decremental V–A conduction can be seen (also in this case, an inverse correlation with the preceding V–V cycle length is shown); the site of earliest atrial activation is most frequently at the CS os/posteroseptal right atrium, and induction with both atrial and ventricular extrastimuli can be obtained.
- However, concerning this case, (a) the AH interval during tachycardia is excessively long to characterize a 'fast' antegrade limb conduction; (b) during fast/slow AVNRT, cycle length variations are caused by higher variability in slow pathway retrograde conduction, so that atrial retrograde activation comes first (A–A change) and V–V changing follows.

- A long R–P tachycardia due to AVRT associated with a concealed decremental posteroseptal accessory pathway, especially in a child, accomplishes the characteristics of PJRT, so that is the most likely diagnosis. Also the mode of repetitive initiation (without any extrastimulus and without any noticeable A–H delay) is compatible with the incessant character of PJRT.

Nonetheless, a definite diagnosis (including differentiation with slow/slow AVNRT) requires further confirmation (e.g. resetting with V stimulation, His refractory ventricular stimulation, V entrainment).

References

1. Heidbuchel H, Jackman WM. Characterization of subforms of AV nodal reentrant tachycardia. *Europace* 2004; **6**: 316–29.

2. Crawford TC, Mukerji S, Good E, *et al*. Utility of atrial and ventricular cycle length variability in determining the mechanism of paroxysmal supraventricular tachycardia. *J Cardiovasc Electrophysiol* 2007; **18**: 698–703.

3. Katritsis DG, Camm AJ. Atrioventricular nodal reentrant tachycardia. *Circulation* 2010; **122**: 831–84.

Introduction to the case

Case 32 focuses on a woman aged 48. After perimitral atrial flutter ablation (Figure 32.1), by means of a linear ablation along the anterior left atrial wall, running from the roof line of the block (box lesion) to the mitral anterior annulus, some pacing (Figure 32.2) manoeuvres were performed in order to validate the isthmus block.

Figure 32.1 Electro-anatomical activation map of the left atrium with the deployed radiofrequency lesions (red tags).

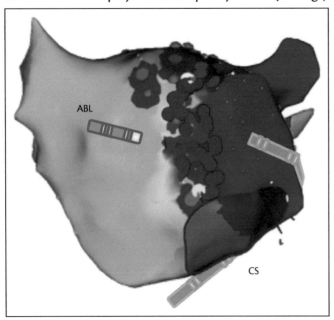

Figure 32.2 Surface lead V1 and intracardiac recordings from the distal to proximal bipoles of the CS and distal and proximal bipoles of the ablation catheter (ABL). Abl: roving mapping catheter into the left atrium (position indicated in figure); ∏: pacing site

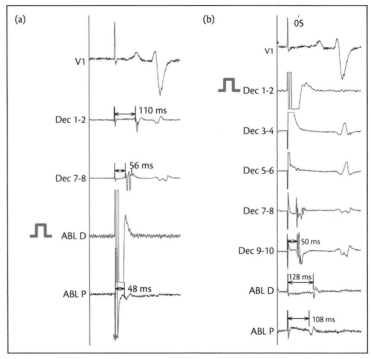

Question

Which of the following is true?

A Both clockwise and counterclockwise blocks are present

B There is clockwise block, but still counterclockwise conduction is present

C There is counterclockwise block, but still clockwise conduction is present

D Bidirectional residual conduction across the ablation line is present

E Validation of bidirectional block needs confirmation with differential pacing

Answer

A **Both clockwise and counterclockwise blocks are present**

Explanation

Pacing to validate block over an ablation line

Pacing from the tip of the mapping catheter (Figure 32.3a) is followed by activation of the proximal dipole and proximal CS, and at last distal CS (positioned next to the line); this implies clockwise conduction block (and not only delay) across the ablation line.[1]

Conversely, pacing from the distal CS (Figure 32.3b) is followed by activation of the proximal CS; the anterior wall is activated late after the CS, from septal to lateral. This is consistent with counterclockwise block (and not only delay) across the ablation line.[1]

References

1. Jais P, Hocini M, Hsu LF, *et al*. Techniques and results of linear ablation at the mitral isthmus. *Circulation* 2004; **110**: 2996–3002.

Figure 32.3 (a) Mapping catheter. (b) Distal CS

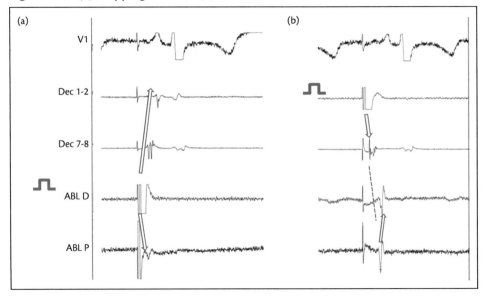

Introduction to the case

This case describes electrogram recordings from a 57-year-old woman (Figure 33.1) during control of PV isolation of the left superior PV (LSPV), using a 10-pole non-irrigated circular ablation and mapping catheter (PVAC) positioned deep inside the PV. Electrograms show pacing of A5 (bipolar pacing from PVAC electrodes 9/10).

Figure 33.1 Bipolar electrograms from a 10-pole ablation catheter. CS: coronary sinus catheter

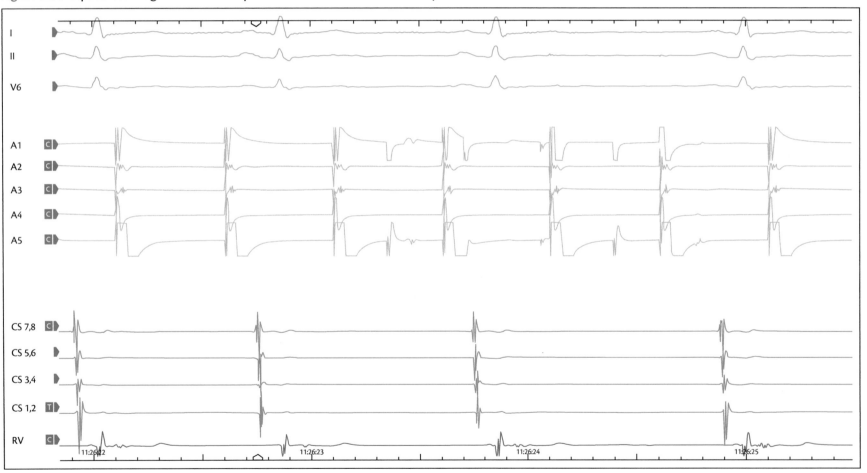

Question

The electrogram proves:

A   PV entrance block

B   Far-field electrograms

C   Far-field capture

D   PV exit block

E   Left atrial appendage dissociation

Answer

D **PV exit block**

Explanation

Exit block from an isolated left superior pulmonary vein

The electrogram shows high-output pacing of the circular mapping catheter deep inside the LSPV. Local (near-field) capture is indicated by the electrograms following each PV-pacing stimulus. No conduction to the left atrium can be identified, indicating local capture of the PV myocardial sleeves with exit block. Indeed, the P-waves are compatible with sinus rhythm.

Exit block evaluation may be a helpful tool with single-shot radiofrequency ablation devices if interpretation of the entrance block may be unclear.[1–3] Usually single-shot radiofrequency ablation devices (like PVAC or nMARQ) have larger electrodes, compared to a regular circular mapping catheter, and far-field electrogram components need to be interpreted more carefully.

References

1. Nentwich K, Duytshaever M, Deneke T. Pulmonary vein isolation: does bidirectional conduction block matter? *Herzschritttmacherther Elektrophysiol* 2014; **25**: 121–2.

2. Duytschaever M, De Meyer G, Acena M, *et al.* Lessons from dissociated pulmonary vein potentials: entry block implies exit block. *Europace* 2013; **15**: 805–12.

3. Vijayaraman P, Dandamudi G, Naperkoski A, Oren J, Storm R, Ellenbogen KA. Assessment of exit block following pulmonary vein isolation: far-field capture masquerading as entrance without exit block. *Heart Rhythm* 2012; **9**: 1653–9.

Introduction to the case

This case describes differential pacing during PV isolation. The Lasso catheter is positioned in the LSPV (Figures 34.1, 34.2, and 34.3).

Figure 34.1 SR

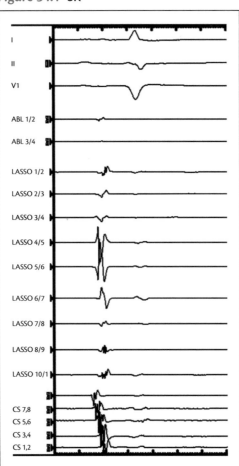

Figure 34.2 Distal CS pace

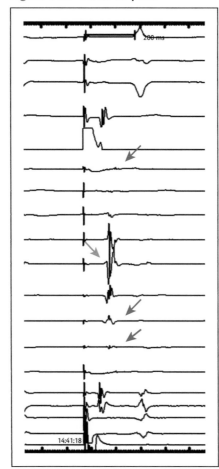

Figure 34.3 LAA pace

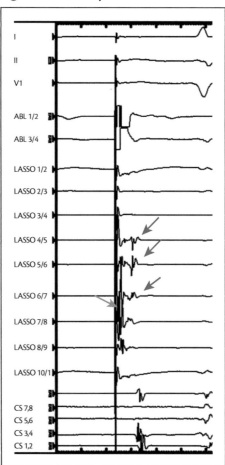

SR: sinus rhythm; LAA: left atrial appendage; Abl: ablation/mapping catheter; Lasso: circular mapping catheter inside the LSPV; CS: coronary sinus catheter

Question

In these tracings, differential pacing is used to:

A   Differentiate local from near-field electrograms

B   Differentiate PV exit block

C   Induce atrial fibrillation

D   Prove entrance block

E   Eliminate near-field capture

Answer

A **Differentiate local from near-field electrograms**

Explanation

Differentiating left atrial appendage and left superior pulmonary vein potentials

Pacing of the CS and the left atrial appendage via the ablation catheter is used to differentiate local PV from far-field electrograms. During sinus rhythm, a multicomponent ('confluent') electrogram is recorded in the LSPV. During distal CS pacing, the left atrial far-field signals (blue arrow) are drawn in towards the pacing spike, allowing for differentiation of far-field and local electrogram components (red arrows). Pacing of the site of the far-field electrogram origin (left atrial appendage usually in the case of the LSPV) allows further differentiation of far-field (blue arrow) and local electrograms (red arrows). The far-field electrogram component is drawn in towards the left atrial appendage pacing spike and the PV potential component spreads out.

Introduction to the case

Case 35 shows an 18-year-old man having palpitations during volleyball. Figure 35.1a
shows S1S2 interval of 410ms during regular pacing at the high right atrium (S1S1 600ms),
and Figure 35.1b shows S1S2 interval of 400ms during regular pacing at the high right
atrium (S1S1 600ms).

Figure 35.1 (a) S1S2 interval of 410ms. (b) S1S2 interval of 400ms. Surface leads I, II, aVF, and V1, and intracardiac recordings from the high right atrium (HRA), the proximal and distal bipoles of the His bundle (HB), the proximal and distal bipoles of the coronary sinus (CS), and the right ventricular apex (RVA). AH: atrio-His interval; CL: cycle length of tachycardia

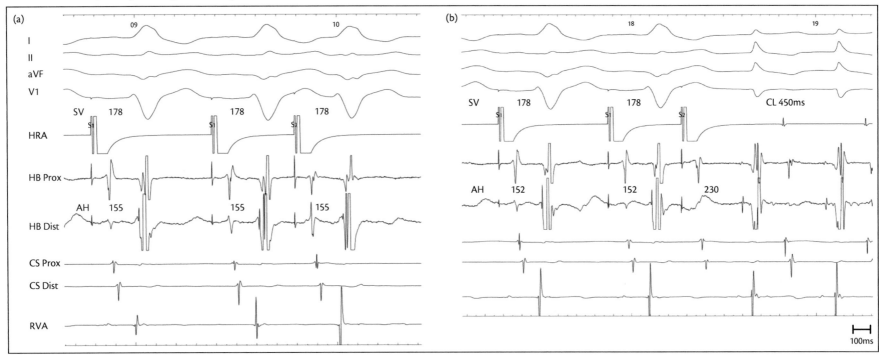

Question

The mechanism of tachycardia (panel b) is:

A   Atypical AVNRT in a patient with LBBB

B   Ectopic right AT in a patient with LBBB

C   AVNRT in a patient with a slow-conducting right-sided bypass tract

D   Orthodromic AVRT using a slow-conducting right-sided bypass tract

E   BBRVT

Answer

D Orthodromic AVRT using a slow-conducting right-sided bypass tract

Explanation

Slow-conducting right-sided bypass tract

Figure 35.1a: during regular pacing at the high right atrium (S1S1 600ms), the QRS complex is characterized by a broad V1-negative and lead I-positive QRS complex. The onset of QRS precedes His bundle activation (negative HV interval). Together with the short *local* HV interval at the His bundle electrogram, this is indicative of the presence of a right-sided bypass tract. The presence of an isoelectric PR segment with a relatively long stimulus-to-onset QRS (S–δ of 178ms), despite pacing nearby the bypass tract and despite the short *local* HV, suggests the presence of a slow anterograde conducting bypass tract. After introducing an S2 stimulus with a coupling interval of 410ms, the QRS morphology is unchanged (i.e. maximal pre-excitation). Also the S–δ interval (178ms) is unchanged. One observation though warrants further clarification—why does the A–H interval remain fixed at 155ms despite prematurity of the extrastimulus (why is the A–H interval not decremental)?

Figure 35.1b: after introducing an S2 stimulus with a coupling interval of 400ms, the bypass tract is refractory (no pre-excitation) and the atrium is conducted to the ventricle using a slow nodal pathway. Apparently, the prolongation of the A–H interval from 152ms to 230ms can be explained by a block in the fast nodal pathway (jump). Slow anterograde conduction over the slow pathway allows retrograde conduction via the right-sided bypass tract, with subsequent initiation of an orthodromic AVRT. The activation at the high right atrium (early compared to the CS and His, but late compared to QRS, VA 190ms) is compatible with orthodromic AVRT via the slow-conducting and right-sided bypass tract. One other puzzling observation still needs further clarification—what is the likelihood of the unique event that an extrastimulus blocks at the same coupling interval both in the fast nodal pathway and the bypass tract?

The present findings are compatible with a slow-conducting right-sided bypass tract with both anterograde and retrograde conduction. During the narrow complex tachycardia and the S2 of 400ms, there is clear proximal-to-distal activation of the His bundle. In contrast, during regular pacing and the S2 of 410ms (maximal pre-excitation), there is distal-to-proximal His bundle activation (Figure 35.2a and

b). This is indicative of retrograde His bundle activation. This explains the fixed A–H interval of 155ms (the A–H interval is determined by the accessory pathway, and not by the anterograde His bundle activation via the node). The hypothesis of retrograde His bundle activation also allows us to explain the initiation of the tachycardia by one single event only during the S2 of 400ms, i.e. block at the bypass tract with unmasking of block at the fast nodal pathway (already present but concealed during regular pacing and an S2 of 410ms). The right-sided bypass tract might be an atrio-fascicular or a 'Mahaim' pathway. Whereas bidirectional conduction and absence of decremental properties (Figure 35.2a and b) is atypical for an atrio-fascicular pathway, some features are typical for a Mahaim fibre: little or no pre-excitation at rest, isoelectric S–δ interval at maximal pre-excitation, typical left bundle branch morphology without slurring, retrograde His bundle activation, and a Mahaim potential with late V at the tricuspid annulus (not shown).

Further explanation

The concept of a right-sided accessory pathway with retrograde His bundle activation is further illustrated during slower regular pacing (S1S1 800ms) (Figure 35.2).

Figure 35.2a: during regular pacing at the high right atrium (S1S1 800ms), the QRS complex is characterized by a fused QRS complex (less pre-excited than in panels (a) and (b)). The His bundle, like during tachycardia, is now activated from proximal to distal (A–H interval during anterograde fast nodal conduction of 120ms). Discrete pre-excitation despite pacing at the high right atrium (near the atrial insertion of the bypass tract) is compatible with the slow-conducting properties of the bypass tract. After introducing an S2 stimulus with a coupling interval of 580ms, pre-excitation is again maximal. Now there is retrograde distal-to-proximal activation of the His bundle, again with an A–H interval of 152ms (identical to that during regular pacing in panels (a) and (b)). Most likely, there is a block of the anterograde fast nodal pathway at this coupling interval (concealed block).

Figure 35.2b: after introducing an S2 stimulus with a coupling interval of 570ms, there is again maximal pre-excitation and the A–H interval remains fixed despite a greater prematurity of the extrastimulus. Again this is compatible with retrograde activation of the His bundle via the bypass tract.

Retrograde His bundle activation has been well described during atrial pacing in patients with a left lateral bypass tract. In the atrio-fascicular accessory pathway (Mahaim pathway), the distal insertion of the bypass tract (into the right bundle) allows retrograde His bundle activation, characterized by a fixed and short V–H interval. Also the relatively early activation of the RV apical electrogram, compared to the delta wave on the surface electrogram, is compatible with an atrio-fascicular, rather than a slowly conducting right free wall AV, pathway.

Anterograde decremental properties of the atrio-fascicular pathway (fixed S-δ with increased pre-excitation) were not observed, most likely because of the relatively late coupled premature beats. The patient was successfully ablated at the tricuspid annulus (7 o' clock) where a clear Mahaim potential was recorded. After delivering radiofrequency energy (and elimination of the accessory pathway), there was anterograde nodal conduction with VA block. Bidirectionally conducting Mahaim fibres (with orthodromic AVRT) have been described.

The hypotheses of a 'non-Mahaim' slow-conducting right-sided bypass tract or the coexistence of an anterograde atrio-fascicular pathway together with a retrograde neighbouring Kent bundle cannot be ruled out but is difficult to accept due to the ablation effect.

Figure 35.2 (a) S1S2 interval of 580ms during regular pacing at the high right atrium (S1S1 800ms). (b) S1S2 interval of 570ms during regular pacing at the high right atrium (S1S1 800ms). Surface leads I, II, aVF, and V1, and intracardiac recordings from the high right atrium (HRA), the proximal and distal bipoles of the His bundle (HB), the proximal and distal bipoles of the coronary sinus (CS), and the right ventricular apex (RVA). AH: atrio-His interval, S-δ: stimulus-to-onset QRS

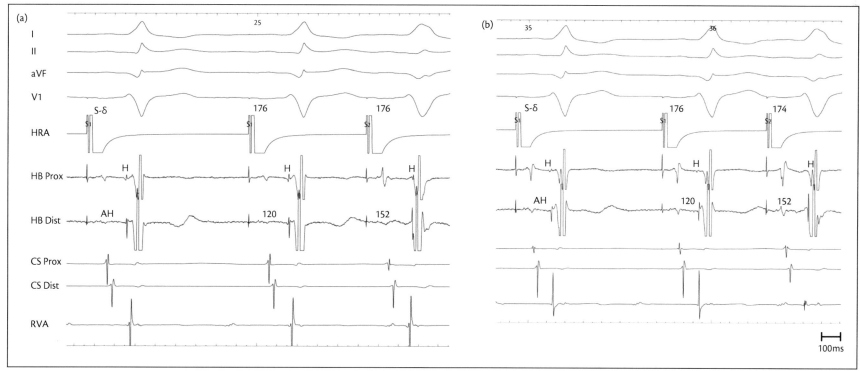

CASE 35

141

Introduction to the case

Case 36 sees a 27-year-old woman with no structural heart disease. Initiation of continuous pacing (300ms) from the RV apex during narrow QRS tachycardia (325ms) is shown in Figure 36.1.

Figure 36.1 Surface leads II, III, and V1, and intracardiac recordings from the distal bipole of the His bundle (HB), the proximal, mid, and distal bipoles of the coronary sinus (CS), and the right ventricular apex (RVA). 'HB' Dist: recording at the distal tip of the His bundle catheter in a too distal position; CS: coronary sinus; RVA: right ventricular apex

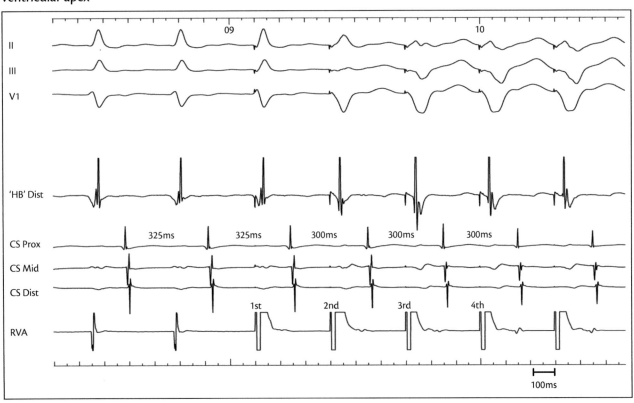

Question

This pacing manoeuvre shows:

A Overdrive of right AT

B Entrainment of fast/slow AVNRT

C Entrainment of orthodromic AVRT

D Overdrive of septal AT

E Inconclusive pacing manoeuvre

143

Answer

C **Entrainment of orthodromic AVRT**

Explanation

Orthodromic atrioventricular re-entrant tachycardia

During continuous ventricular pacing, tachycardia is entrained starting from the 2nd paced beat (the 1st paced beat does not conduct to the atrium, no reset). Apparently (limited number of electrodes), atrial activation seems unaltered during pacing. This observation reduces the likelihood of AT (with the exception of low septal origin).

The QRS morphology of the 2nd paced beat is different from the 3rd, 4th, etc. beat. Nevertheless, the atrial activation following this 2nd paced beat is already reset (advanced). In this setting, the QRS morphology change is a sign of progressive and manifest fusion. Reset of the atrium together with fusion can only happen in AVRT (fusion between the orthodromic wavefront of AVRT and part of the ventricle activated by pacing).

In case of entrainment of AVNRT or overdrive of AT, fusion between intrinsic AV conduction and ventricular pacing may occur as well, but once the atrium is reset, the QRS complex preceding (and following) the 1st reset atrium can only have a 'pure' paced morphology.

In this patient, the bypass tract was located and successfully ablated at the tricuspid annulus (12 o' clock).

Note: the fact that a late-coupled 'premature beat' from the RV apex (His refractoriness can be assumed despite the absence of a clear His bundle recording) advances the atrium is compatible with a right-sided bypass tract.

Introduction to the case

This case presents counterclockwise mitral flutter that slowed during mitral isthmus ablation (from 232 to 251ms) but that did not terminate despite extensive ablation (Figure 37.1). A remap of the flutter (cycle length 251ms) revealed the correct diagnosis (Figure 37.2).

Figure 37.1 Mitral flutter slowed during mitral isthmus ablation from 232 to 251ms

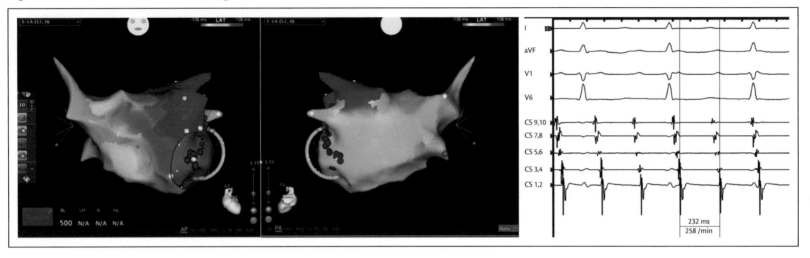

Figure 37.2 A remap of the flutter (cycle length 251ms) revealed the correct diagnosis

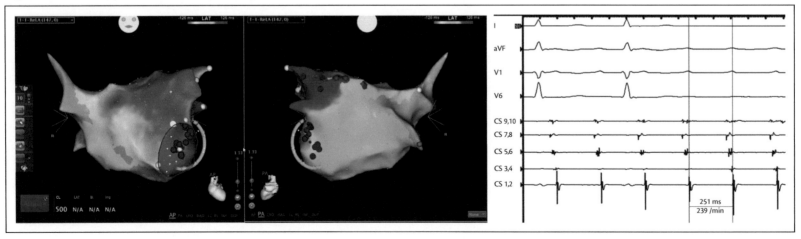

Question

What is the mechanism of the tachycardia (cycle length 251ms)?

A   AT from the LSPV

B   Atrial tachycardia around the mitral isthmus

C   Atrial tachycardia involving the CS

D   Atrial tachycardia involving another epicardial structure

E   None of the above

Answer

D   Atrial tachycardia involving another epicardial structure

Explanation

Perimitral flutter, or is it?

In Figure 37.2, the latest activation is seen near the upper part of the posterior left atrium. Therefore, the flutter does not involve the CS as an epicardial structure, which is situated at the lower left atrium in the AV groove. The only anatomical structure going from the ridge between the LSPV and the appendage is the ligament of Marshall, which inserts in the mid-posterior CS and can serve as an electrical conduit refractory to endocardial radiofrequency application. This is proven during contrast injection of the vein that led to conversion of the tachycardia

(Figure 37.3), and by pacing from the left atrial appendage (Figure 37.4). Ethanol injection into the vein of Marshall could induce complete isthmus block over the mitral isthmus (Figure 37.4, lower panel).

In this case the flutter terminated during contrast injection into the vein of Marshall using a right coronary catheter (Figure 37.3). Mitral conduction was demonstrated by pacing in the left atrial appendage (Figure 37.4 a). After ethanol injection into the vein of Marshall (1cc, two injections), mitral block was demonstrated (Figure 37.4b).

Figure 37.3 Flutter converted during contrast injection into the vein of Marshall

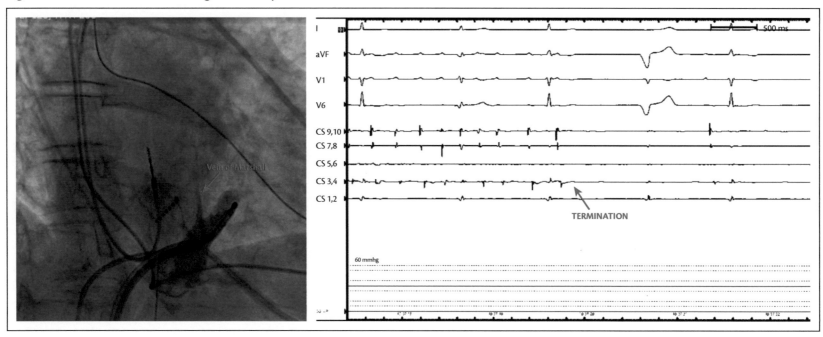

Figure 37.4 (a) Mitral conduction was demonstrated by pacing in the left atrial appendage. (b) After ethanol injection into the vein of Marshall (1cc, two injections), mitral block was demonstrated. Ethanol injection into the vein of Marshall has been proved to facilitate mitral block.

Reproduced from José L. Báez-Escudero *et al*, ethanol infusion in the vein of Marshall facilitates mitral isthmus ablation. *Heart Rhythm*. 2012 Vol. 9, No. 8 with permission from Elsevier

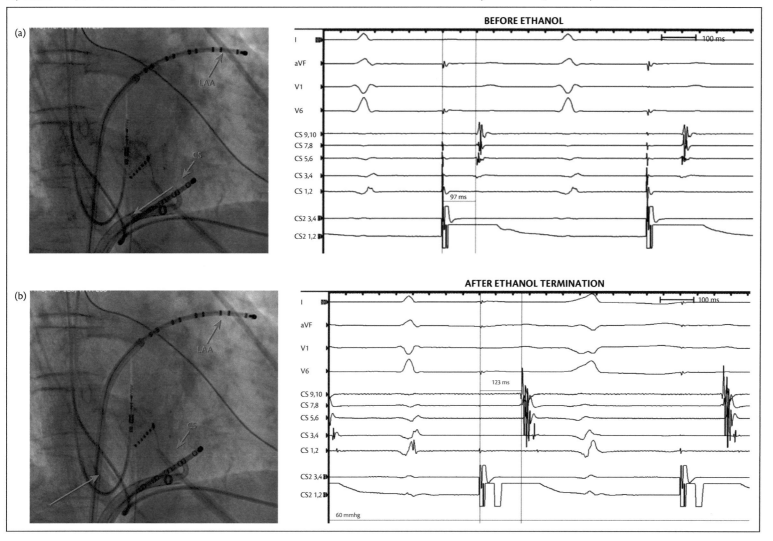

Introduction to the case

After continuation of induced tachycardia for more than a minute, the following manoeuvre (Figure 38.1) is performed on a woman aged 17.

Figure 38.1 Pacing manoeuvre during narrow QRS tachycardia. RAA: right atrial appendage; HBp till HBd: His bundle recordings from proximal to distal; PS: posteroseptal recording; CS: coronary sinus; A: atrial electrogram; H: His bundle deflection; S: stimulus

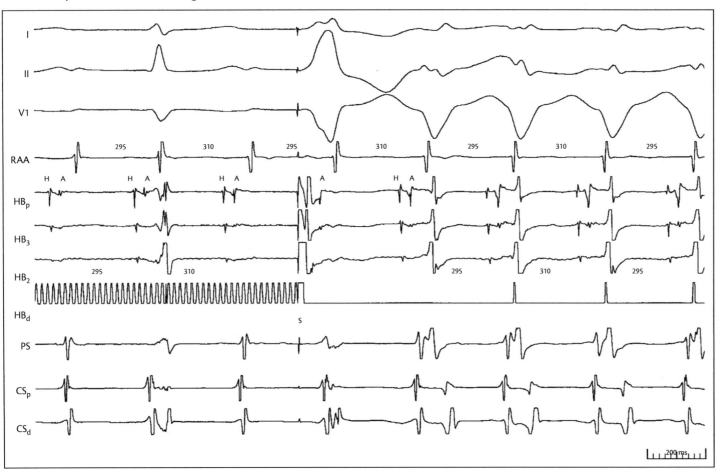

Question

Which statement describes best what happens during the recording?

A   A ventricular extrastimulus induces Mahaim tachycardia

B   A ventricular extrastimulus induces AVNRT

C   A ventricular extrastimulus induces bundle branch re-entrant tachycardia

D   A ventricular extrastimulus recruits distal right bundle branch conduction

E   A ventricular extrastimulus induces distal LBBB

Answer

D **A ventricular extrastimulus recruits distal right bundle branch conduction**

Explanation

A single ventricular extrastimulus during supraventricular tachycardia/2

The 2:1 block in this patient with AVNRT is clearly infra-His, since a proximal potential is still present. There must be a concomitant block in the distal right and left bundles to explain the 2:1 AV block. A ventricular extrastimulus (S) is delivered from the tip of the His bundle catheter, i.e. stimulating the proximal interventricular septum. There is no direct capture of the His bundle/right bundle itself, proven by the early retrograde activation of the right bundle that can be seen shortly after the stimulus artefact in HB2 (Figure 38.2).[1] (Note also that there is retrograde conduction to the atrium, with the same atrial activation sequence, which makes AT highly unlikely.) The premature retrograde activation of the right bundle (305ms) leads to the subsequent lengthening of the H–H interval (315ms) which is just enough to enable resumption of 1:1 conduction over the right bundle (but with persistent LBBB). This leads to a shortening of the distal right bundle activation (now at ± 300ms vs ± 600ms in the initial part of the tracing). The shortened activation leads also to a shortening of the distal right bundle refractory period, which explains the ensuing 1:1 conduction in the right bundle. While at the left of the tracing there was a simultaneous 2:1 block in both bundle branches, now the right bundle regained 1:1 conduction. The same phenomenon did not occur in the left bundle (pacing was delivered on the right side). Moreover, also concealed retrograde penetration of the left bundle will maintain persistent LBBB.

Figure 38.2 provides some further explanation.

Figure 38.2 Same figure as Figure 38.1, but with added annotations. RAA: right atrial appendage; HBp till HBd: His bundle recordings from proximal to distal; PS: posteroseptal recording; CS: coronary sinus; A: atrial electrogram; H: His bundle deflection; S: stimulus

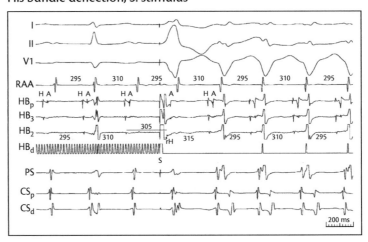

References

1. Heidbuchel H, Jackman WM. Characterization of subforms of AV nodal reentrant tachycardia. *Europace* 2004; **6**: 316–29.

Introduction to the case

The patient, a woman aged 59, was admitted for ablation of circus movement tachycardia over a left anterolateral accessory pathway. A mapping and ablation catheter (Figure 39.1) is introduced into the left atrium via a trans-septal sheath and positioned at two positions, 2mm apart, alongside the mitral annulus during ventricular pacing (Figure 39.2) from a para-Hisian position.

Figure 39.1 A mapping and ablation catheter is introduced into the left atrium via a trans-septal sheath and positioned at two positions, 2 mm apart, alongside the mitral annulus during ventricular pacing

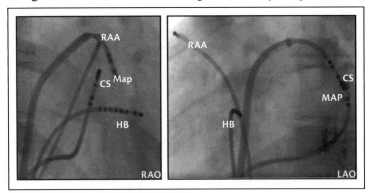

Figure 39.2 Electrograms on the mapping catheter at the two positions alongside the mitral annulus during ventricular pacing. RAA: right atrial appendage; HBp till HBd: His bundle recordings from proximal to distal; Map: mapping catheter (bipolar electrogram); CS: coronary sinus; H: His bundle deflection; S: stimulus

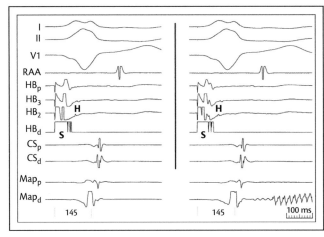

Question

A mapping and ablation catheter is introduced into the left atrium via a trans-septal sheath and positioned alongside the mitral annulus during ventricular pacing from a para-Hisian position. At which position would you ablate?

A   Based on the electrogram in Figure 39.3a

B   Based on the electrogram in Figure 39.3b

Figure 39.3a

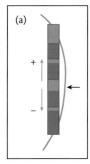

Figure 39.3b

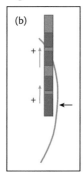

Answer

B   Based on the electrogram in Figure 39.3b

Explanation

Electrograms during accessory pathway ablation

The timing of the earliest atrial activation on the ablation bipole (Map d) is similar in both panels. The atrial electrograms are smaller than the ventricular electrograms, as is desired for ablation. In the left panel, there is a clear polarity reversal of the atrial electrograms, being initially positive in the proximal mapping bipole and negative in the distal bipole. This indicates that the insertion of the accessory pathway is located in the middle between both bipoles. Delivering energy from the 4mm ablation tip would be too inferior in relation to the insertion and hence would fail to ablate the accessory pathway. At the right side, the catheter tip has been withdrawn a few millimetres more towards the anterior mitral annulus. The timing of the earliest atrial activation is the same, but there is now a small initial positive deflection on the distal ablation bipole. Therefore, the ablation tip now resides over the atrial insertion of the accessory pathway itself. Such finely titrated ablation position will usually lead to a block of the accessory pathway conduction within a few seconds after initiation of energy delivery.

Figure 39.4 helps to explain further.

Figure 39.4 Same figures as Figures 39.1 and 39.2, but with extra annotations. RAA: right atrial appendage; HBp till HBd: His bundle recordings from proximal to distal; CS: coronary sinus; Map: mapping catheter; A: atrial electrogram; H: His bundle deflection; S: stimulus

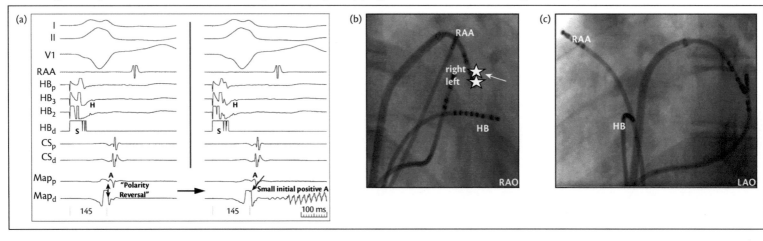

Introduction to the case

During His catheter insertion for a diagnostic electrophysiological study, the following tachycardia (Figure 40.1) was observed. What is the tachycardia mechanism?

Figure 40.1 Surface ECG leads; HRA: high right atrium

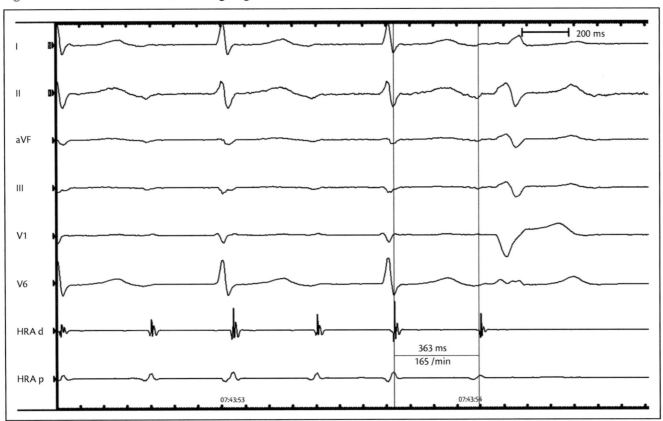

Question

The correct diagnosis is:

A   Atrial tachycardia with 2:1 AV block

B   Atrial flutter with 2:1 conduction

C   AVNRT

D   Orthodromic reciprocating tachycardia (ORT)

E   Other

Answer

C **AVNRT**

Explanation

A ventricular bump during supraventricular tachycardia

This case illustrates that electrophysiological workout should start already at the beginning of the procedure (even in the presence of a minimal amount of catheters). Orthodromic AV re-entry tachycardia is excluded, because more atrial than ventricular activations are present.[1] The SVT has a rate of 166/min (cycle length of 363ms), which is unusual for right-sided flutter. Atrial tachycardia (AV) (originating from the lower septum, see narrow negative P-waves) with 2:1 conduction could be possible. Two observations speak against this hypothesis: (1) the 2:1 fixed block with an AV interval of 360ms and the AV node very poorly conducting with only 720ms cycle length of the RR interval. One would rather expect Wenckebach-type prolongation and blocking in the AV node at this rate; (2) in addition, termination by a ventricular extrasystole without affecting atrial activation makes AT almost impossible. The termination then would not be caused by premature depolarization of tissue surrounding the focus, but only by an increase in atrial pressure caused by the PVC. This is known, but rare.

The most likely mechanism is AVNRT with 2:1 block in the lower common pathway (LCP) or 2:1 intra- or infra-His block, caused by mechanical block during His catheter insertion.[1] The mechanism of termination is concealed conduction into the slow pathway of the AV node, rendering this part of the re-entry circuit refractory for the next tachycardia beat.

The tachycardia was easily inducible during the electrophysiological study with frequent LCP block and became non-inducible after ablation of the slow pathway.

References

1. Knight BP1, Ebinger M, Oral H, *et al*. Diagnostic value of tachycardia features and pacing maneuvers during paroxysmal supraventricular tachycardia. *J Am Coll Cardiol* 2000; **36**: 574–82.

Introduction to the case

This case discusses a 46-year-old woman with corrected Graves' hyperthyroidism (Figure 41.1).

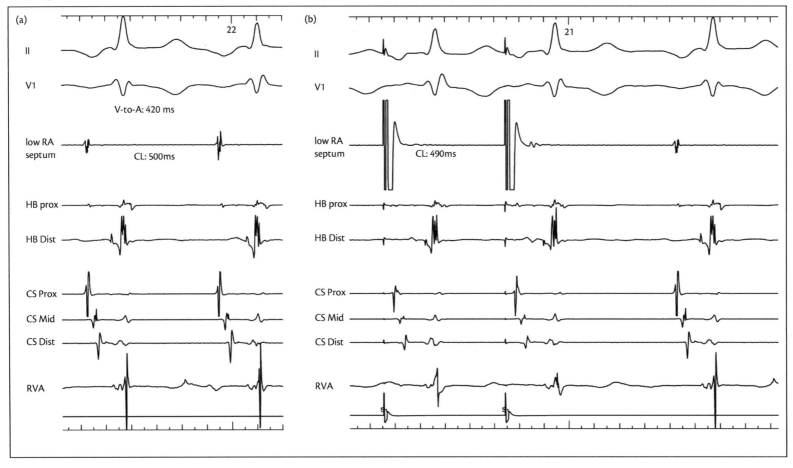

Figure 41.1 (a) Slow tachycardia (cycle length, CL = 500ms) with long VA interval. (b) Atrial overdrive pacing (CL = 490ms) was performed, after which the tachycardia continued. Surface leads II and V1 and intracardiac recordings from the ablation catheter at the low right atrial (RA) septum, His bundle (HB), coronary sinus (CS), and right ventricular apex (RVA)

Question

The underlying mechanism of the tachycardia is:

A Atypical AVNRT

B Fascicular VT

C AT

D Orthodromic AVRT using a slow-conducting accessory pathway (PJRT)

E Inconclusive pacing manoeuvre

Answer

C AT

Explanation

Atrial tachycardia

The patient has a long RP tachycardia (V-to-A interval of 420ms) with a negative P-wave in the inferior leads. Together with atrial activation being earlier at the low right atrial septum than at the His bundle region, this could be explained by atypical AVNRT (fast/slow), orthodromic AVRT using a slow-conducting posteroseptal bypass tract (PJRT), or septal AT.

Upon cessation of atrial overdrive pacing, tachycardia continues. The V-to-A interval of the return cycle (525ms) is markedly longer than the V-to-A interval during tachycardia (420ms). A variable V-to-A interval (difference in V-to-A of >14ms) suggests atrial tachycardia. In AVNRT or orthodromic AVRT, the V-to-A interval is expected to be fixed (difference within 10ms) because the timing of atrial activation is dependent on ventricular activation (VA linking).

In the present case, the diagnosis of AT was confirmed and successfully ablated.

Note: in AT, one can observe a fixed V-to-A interval if pacing is performed next to the focus (with a short return cycle). To reduce this ambiguity, it is better to pace remote from the site of earliest activation or to pace from two sites.

Note: in AVNRT or PJRT, a variable V-to-A interval can be observed in the case of pacing-induced decremental VA conduction. To reduce this ambiguity, it is essential to pace the atrium only slightly faster than the tachycardia rate. In the present case, it seems unlikely that shortening of the atrial cycle length by 10ms would account for a decrement in VA conduction of >100ms.

Introduction to the case

The patient, a 65-year-old male, underwent catheter ablation for paroxysmal atrial fibrillation, aiming at circumferential PV isolation (PVI). Electrogram recordings during circumferential ablation of the left-sided PVs are shown (Figure 42.1). Radiofrequency delivery is started anteriorly at the ridge in between the LSPV and left atrial appendage.

Figure 42.1 Electrogram recording during ablation of the left-sided PVs. The circular mapping catheter is positioned in the LSPV. LASSO: circular PV mapping catheter; Abl EIN: onset of radiofrequency delivery; ABL: ablation catheter; CS: coronary sinus catheter

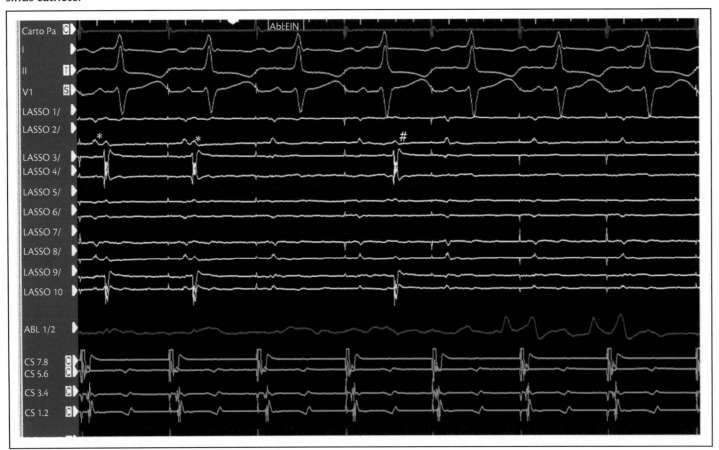

Question

What happens after onset of ablation?

A   Occurrence of dissociated PV activity

B   Occurrence of PV exit block

C   Occurrence of PV entrance block

D   PV tachycardia

E   Far-field oversensing

Answer

C Occurrence of PV entrance block

Explanation

Isolation of the left superior pulmonary vein

During the last two beats before ablation, each far-field atrial electrogram is followed by a sharp near-field potential (*) from the PV. This local PV potential disappears instantaneously after onset of ablation, indicating conduction block into the PV (entrance block). The next beat is characterized by resumption of LA–PV conduction, as evidenced by delayed PV potential (#, identical morphology), after which permanent entrance block is observed. Entry block is almost invariably associated with exit block.

The alternative hypothesis that the delayed PV potential (#) is due to spontaneous or dissociated PV activity is unlikely because of the isolated nature of this beat and because of its identical activation pattern compared to entrance conduction.

Introduction to the case

A woman's RSPV is evaluated during ongoing PV ablation. The Lasso catheter (bipolar electrograms) is positioned at the LA–PV junction. Unipolar electrograms are recorded at the SVC (Figure 43.1).

Figure 43.1 Circular mapping (Lasso) catheter recordings positioned at the LA–PV junction of the RSPV. RSPV: right superior pulmonary vein; SVC: superior vena cava; CS: coronary sinus; LAS: Lasso catheter; MAP: mapping catheter

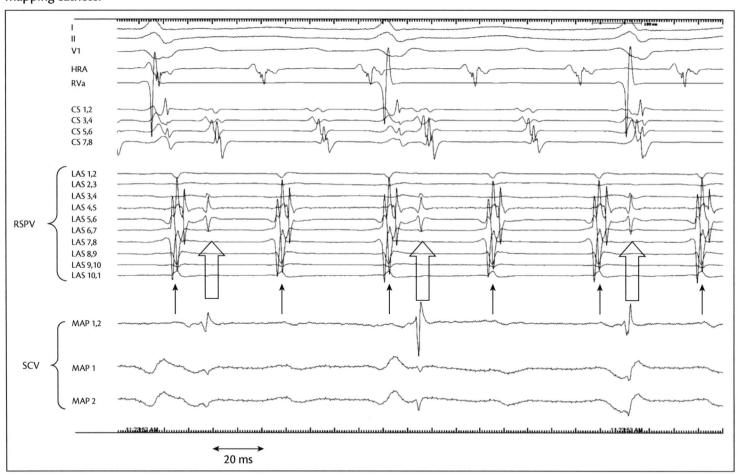

Question

Local electrical activity is recorded with a Lasso catheter in the RSPV during AT (bold arrows).
On Lasso 4-5 and 5-6, deflections are recorded at a slow, regular rate as well (open arrows).
These deflections are caused by:

A   Spontaneous ectopic activity in the PV

B   Activity in the PV triggered by AT-related activation

C   Remote activity in the superior vena cava (SVC) (far-field)

D   Activity in the CS

Answer

C **Remote activity in the superior vena cava (SVC) (far-field)**

Explanation

Far-field superior vena cava potentials recorded from the right superior pulmonary vein

Compared to unipolar recordings, bipolar recordings reduce deflections caused by remote activity more, but not completely. If excitable structures are adjacent, activation in one structure may cause a related deflection in a bipolar electrode positioned in the other structure.[1,2] The SVC is located adjacent to the RSPV (Figure 43.2). Next to atrial tachycardia-induced deflections in the RSPV (bold arrows), additional deflections in the RSPV occur (open arrows) in a 2-to-1 way that coincide with SVC deflections, supporting their SVC origin.[3,4] Such remote deflections in the RSPV (or other PVs) might erroneously be interpreted as failed isolation of the RSPV.

Note: the regular rhythm in the SVC is caused by physiological 2:1 block at the right atrial–SVC junction during AT.

References

1. Brouwer J, Nagelkerke D, den Heijer P, *et al.* Analysis of atrial sensed far-field ventricular signals: a reassessment. *Pacing Clin Electrophysiol* 1997; **20**: 916–22.

2. de Bakker JM, Wittkampf FH. The pathophysiologic basis of fractionated and complex electrograms and the impact of recording techniques on their detection and interpretation. *Circ Arrhythm Electrophysiol* 2010; **3**: 204–13.

3. Ho SY, Cabrera JA, Tran VH, Farre J, Anderson RH, Sanchez-Quintana D. Architecture of the pulmonary veins: relevance to radiofrequency ablation. *Heart* 2001; **86**: 265–70.

4. Hocini M, Ho SY, Kawara T, *et al.* Electrical conduction in canine pulmonary veins: electrophysiological and anatomic correlation. *Circulation* 2002; **105**: 2442–8.

Figure 43.2 The superior vena cava

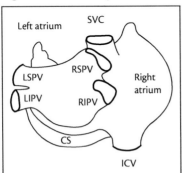

Introduction to the case

A 72-year-old woman with severe dilated cardiomyopathy and cardiac resynchronization therapy defibrillator (CRT-D) implantation had persistent atrial fibrillation with rapid ventricular response. She was scheduled to undergo AV nodal ablation. The ablation catheter was advanced to the level of the cardiac silhouette (Figure 44.1a) but was impossible to advance into the RV and no near-field electrograms were recorded (Figure 44.1b).

Figure 44.1 Procedural findings. (a) The ablation catheter advanced to the level of the cardiac silhouette . (b) Electrogram of the ablation catheter

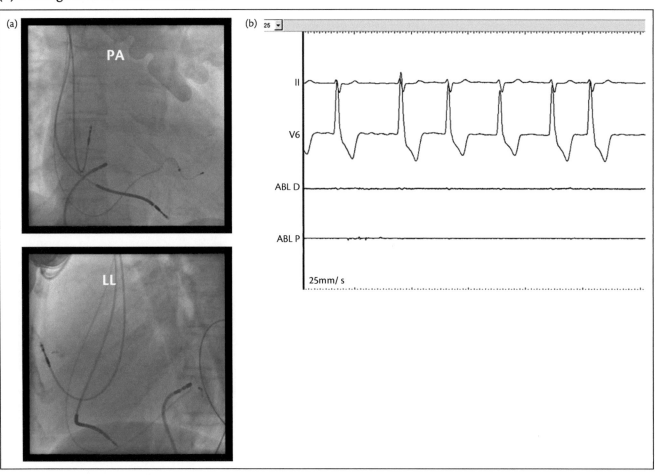

Question

Where is the ablation catheter positioned?

A   Right atrium with atrial standstill

B   Descending aorta

C   Azygos vein

D   Thoracic vein

E   Mediastinal space

Answer

C **Azygos vein**

Explanation

Azygos continuation of an interrupted inferior vena cava

The catheter is too posterior to be in the right atrium (LL view). The descending aorta is posterior, but the catheter would be more to the patient's left in the PA view. This patient has azygos continuation of an interrupted inferior vena cava. This anomaly occurs in 0.8% of the population requiring electrophysiological procedures[1] and is due to agenesis of the hepatic tract of the inferior vena cava. The caudal segment of the inferior vena cava reaches the azygos system via a persistent right supracardinal vein.[2] The anomaly has no functional consequences, other than rendering some ablation procedures difficult via an inferior access (e.g. in case a trans-septal puncture is required). Procedures such as cavotricuspid isthmus ablation or slow pathway modification are, however, relatively easily performed, as was ablation of the AV node in our patient (the position of the catheter advanced into the heart is shown in Figure 44.2).

References

1. Minniti S, Visentini S, Procacci C. Congenital anomalies of the venae cavae: embryological origin, imaging features and report of three new variants. *Eur Radiol* 2002; **12**: 2040–55.
2. Perez-Silva A, Merino JL, Peinado R, Lopez-Sendon J. Atrial flutter ablation through the azygous continuation in a patient with inferior vena cava interruption. *Europace* 2011; **13**: 442–3.

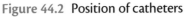

Figure 44.2 Position of catheters

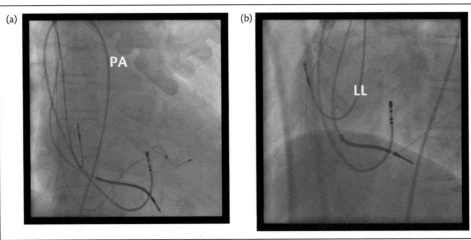

(a) PA (b) LL

Introduction to the case

A 26-year-old woman with a history of SVT underwent an electrophysiological procedure, with repeated induction of a narrow complex tachycardia by premature atrial stimulation. During a diagnostic ventricular overdrive manoeuvre, the tracing (Figure 45.1) in the figure was recorded.

Figure 45.1 Diagnostic RV overdrive pacing manoeuvre performed during tachycardia. Note: The RV channel is saturated by the pacing artefact. RV: right ventricle; HRA p: high right atrium proximal; HRA d: high right atrium distal

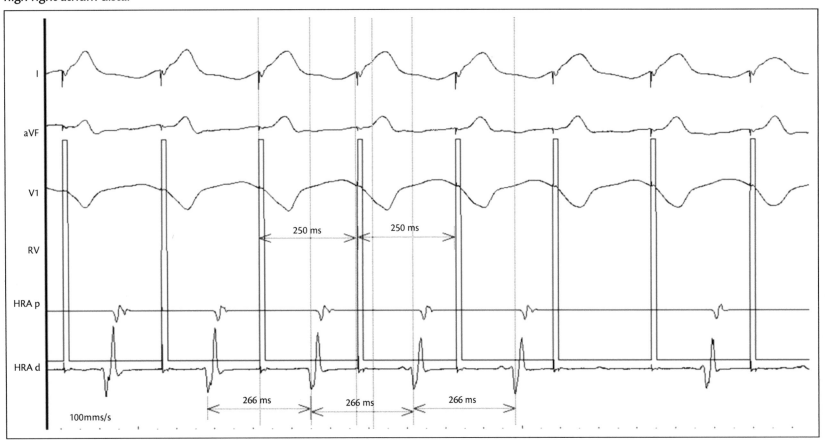

Question

Which of the following statements is true?

A   AT can be excluded

B   AVNRT can be excluded

C   AVRT can be excluded

D   Answers A and C are correct

E   None of the above are correct

Answer

D   Answers A and C are correct

Explanation

Interruption of a supraventricular tachycardia by a ventricular overdrive pacing manoeuvre

The tachycardia is interrupted by ventricular overdrive pacing, without atrial reset, thus ruling out AT.[1] AVRT can be ruled out because there is no consistent retrograde VA conduction. The diagnosis must therefore be AVNRT. Although coincident termination of AT cannot be ruled out entirely, the exact similar atrial activation sequence and electrogram morphology during ventricular pacing as during tachycardia make AT unlikely. In case the tachycardia had been interrupted with atrial reset, the differential diagnosis would have remained AT, AVNRT, or AVRT. AV dissociation during ventricular overdrive pacing without interruption of the tachycardia would have ruled out AVRT.

References

1. Knight BP, Ebinger M, Oral H,*et al.* Diagnostic value of tachycardia features and pacing maneuvers during paroxysmal supraventricular tachycardia. *J Am Coll Cardiol* 2000; **36**: 574–82.

Introduction to the case

Case 46 presents a 58-year-old man who has been referred for catheter ablation of recurrent symptomatic tachycardias. He had a history of inferior wall myocardial infarction (MI) 15 years ago and coronary artery bypass graft 9 years ago. Tracing was recorded (Figure 46.1) during isoproterenol infusion at the end of a train of atrial stimulation with an extrastimulus (230ms; last S at beginning of tracing).

Figure 46.1 Electrophysiological study: pacing during isoproterenol infusion. HIS d: distal His bundle; HIS p: proximal His bundle; HRA: high right atrium; P1 art: arterial line; S: stimulus; H: His; V: ventricle; A: atrium

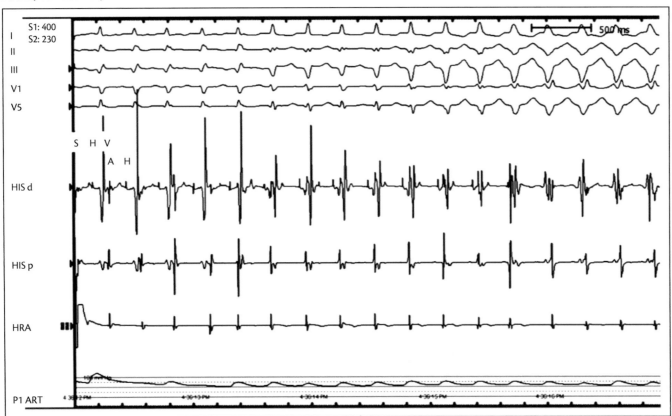

Question

The tracing shows:

A   AVNRT with progressive conduction aberrancy

B   AT with progressive conduction over an accessory pathway

C   Orthodromic tachycardia changing for antidromic tachycardia

D   Fascicular VT

E   SVT inducing VT

Answer

E   **SVT inducing VT**

Explanation

From narrow to wide QRS tachycardia

Under isoproterenol infusion, a train of atrial stimulation with an extrastimulus (230ms) induces a narrow QRS tachycardia.

The differential diagnosis for the narrow QRS tachycardia is AVNRT, AVRT, or AT. Based on the tracing,[1] the diagnosis cannot be definitively determined. Initiation of tachycardia was preceded by only a modest increase in AH interval (from 106 to 146ms), not diagnostic of dual AV nodal pathways. The septal VA time of 75ms is non-diagnostic and is not sufficiently short (e.g. <70ms) to exclude the presence of an accessory pathway. The TCL does oscillate with H–H interval oscillations anticipating AA oscillations in some beats, consistent with involvement of the AV node in the arrhythmia, but the VA time is not fixed, so that fortuitous occurrence of this finding with an AT would be a concern. The high right atrium appears relatively early, but these recordings are from the proximal electrodes that were close to the atrial septum.

The wide QRS tachycardia occurs with gradual fusion between activation over the His–Purkinje system and the ventricles, as evident from a progressive decrease in HV interval until the His is no longer visible. Thus, aberrancy due to bundle branch block is excluded. The absence of pre-excitation during atrial pacing is not in favour of pre-excitation. Mapping and entrainment led to the diagnosis of scar-related VT due to prior MI.

References

1. Sacher F, Vest J, Raymond JM, Stevenson WG. Atrial pacing inducing narrow QRS tachycardia followed by wide complex tachycardia. *J Cardiovasc Electrophysiol* 2007; **18**: 1213–15.

Introduction to the case

Case 47 looks at a woman, aged 42, with recurrent implantable cardioverter–defibrillator (ICD) shocks. She was diagnosed with arrhythmogenic right ventricular cardiomyopathy (ARVC) at age 20. Because of recurrent VT despite beta-blocker therapy, she was implanted with an ICD at age 30. One year ago, she underwent an endocardial VT ablation procedure that was not successful and was therefore referred for epicardial ablation. Pacing (Figure 47.1) from the ablation catheter was 450ms, whereas TCL was 470ms.

Figure 47.1 Pacing manoeuvres. RFd: distal bipole of the ablation catheter; RFp: proximal bipole of the ablation catheter; RVd: distal bipole of the catheter placed at the RV apex; CSd: distal bipole of the catheter placed in the coronary sinus

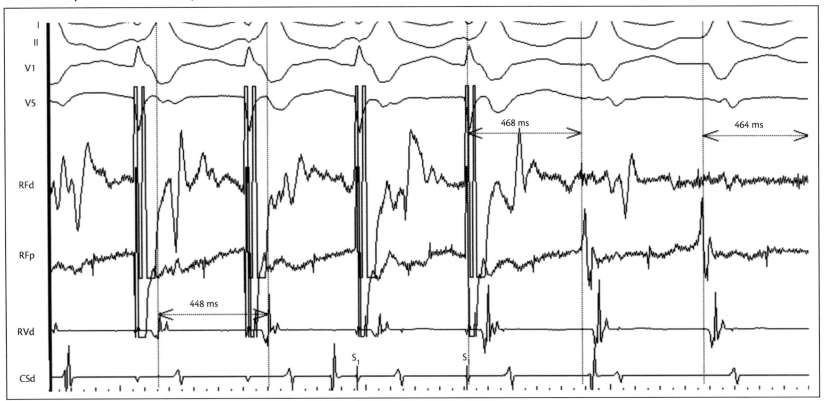

Question

Which part of the VT circuit is paced?

A   Not possible to say since it is not captured

B   The exit of the VT isthmus

C   An outer loop

D   The entrance of the VT isthmus

E   A bystander area

Answer

B   The exit of the VT isthmus

Explanation

Where are we within the ventricular tachycardia circuit?

1. The potential is captured with acceleration of the cycle length (CL) to 448ms (Figure 47.2).
2. The return CL is equal to the TCL; the pacing site is in the circuit.
3. The captured potential is just before the QRS and the S–QRS/VT CL is <30%.
4. The 12-leads is not shown, but the morphology is identical during VT and pacing (concealed fusion), meaning that the pacing site is in the protected area with the same exit site as the VT, even if there is a slight change in V5 (one QRS out of two), possibly indicating a slightly different exit because of the different refractory period of the exit path.
5. Finally, in term of the ablation target, a site where a mid-diastolic potential can be found should be tried first, probably by going more inside the scar.[1-4]

References

1. Stevenson WG, Khan H, Sager P, *et al*. Identification of reentry circuit sites during catheter mapping and radiofrequency ablation of ventricular tachycardia late after myocardial infarction. *Circulation* 1993; **88**: 1647–70.

2. Stevenson WG, Friedman PL, Sager PT, *et al*. Exploring postinfarction reentrant ventricular tachycardia with entrainment mapping. *J Am Coll Cardiol* 1997; **29**: 1180–9.

3. Raymond JM, Sacher F, Winslow R, Tedrow U, Stevenson WG. Catheter ablation for scar-related ventricular tachycardias. *Curr Probl Cardiol* 2009; **34**: 225–70.

4. Josephson ME, Almendral J, Callans DJ. Resetting and entrainment of reentrant ventricular tachycardia associated with myocardial infarction. *Heart Rhythm* 2014; **11**: 1239–49.

Figure 47.2 Entrainment during VT

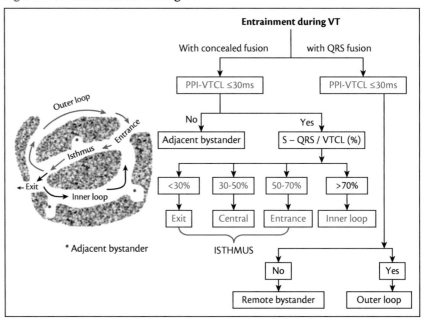

Adapted from Stevenson WG, Friedman PL, Sager PT, Saxon LA, Kocovic D, Harada T, Wiener I, Khan H. Exploring postinfarction reentrant ventricular tachycardia with entrainment mapping. *J Am Coll Cardiol*. 1997 May;29(6):1180–9 with permission from Elsevier.

Introduction to the case

A man, aged 63, with ischaemic and valvular cardiomyopathy (prosthetic mitral valve), left ventricular ejection fraction (LVEF) of 30%, and complete AV block is shown in this case. Figure 48.1a shows an electrogram during pacing with his device (underlying AV block) just before ventricular stimulation. Figure 48.1b shows a train of RV apex stimulation at a cycle length of 600ms with S2/S3 coupling intervals of 240 and 280ms, respectively. The ablation catheter (RFd) is located at the inferior wall of the LV within the scar.

Figure 48.1 (a) Electrogram during pacing before ventricular stimulation. (b) A train of RV apex stimulation at a cycle length of 600ms. RFd: distal bipole of the ablation catheter; RFp: proximal bipole of the ablation catheter; RV 1-2: distal bipole of the catheter placed at the RV apex

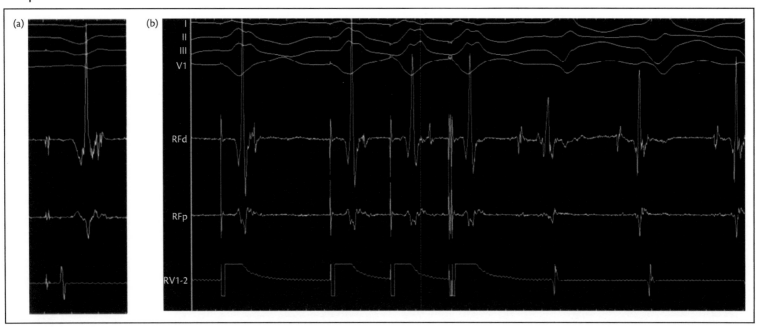

Question

What happens on panel B?

A   Return to device pacing due to underlying AV block

B   Probable local functional delay during S2/S3 in a ventricular scar inducing VT

C   AT induction

D   Antidromic tachycardia induction through an accessory pathway

E   Bundle branch re-entrant tachycardia

Answer

B **Probable local functional delay during S2/S3 in a ventricular scar inducing VT**

Explanation

Pacing manoeuvre during ventricular tachycardia

Figure 48.2 shows the baseline electrogram with a high-frequency, low-voltage signal after the V electrogram that corresponds to poorly coupled ventricular activity (scar area).[1] During RV pacing, the delay between the normal and abnormal electrograms increases and is accentuated with a shorter coupling interval S2, and an important delay (as a jump) occurs on S3 (probable functional conduction delay in the scar area). This is in fact the mechanism responsible for the VT initiation. The sharp low-voltage potential (arrow) is situated just before QRS onset during VT with reversed polarity, compared to pacing train, possibly indicating a reversed activation. Together with entrainment manoeuvres (not shown, but there were concealed fusion and a perfect return cycle length), the catheter was localized between the central part and the exit of the isthmus responsible of this VT.

Figure 48.2 Baseline electrogram with a high-frequency, low-voltage signal

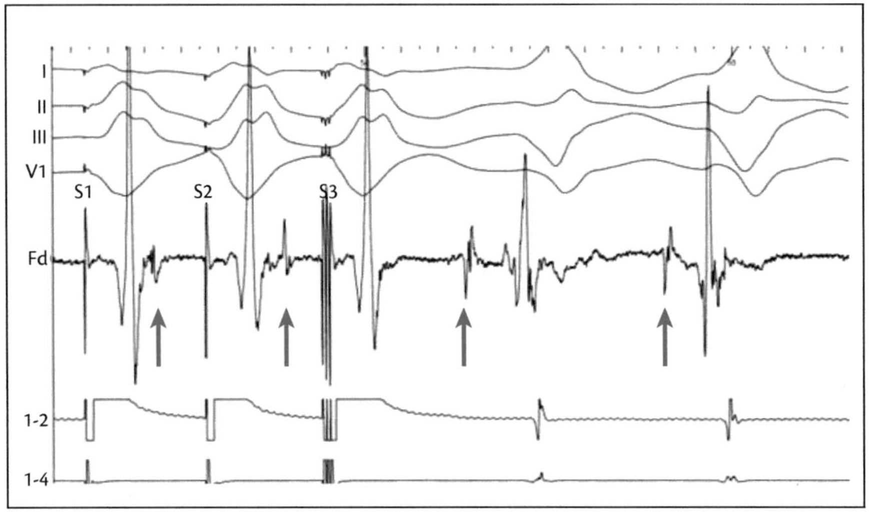

References

1. Jaïs P, Maury P, Khairy P, *et al*. Elimination of local abnormal ventricular activities: a new end point for substrate modification in patients with scar-related ventricular tachycardia. *Circulation* 2012; **125**: 2184–96.

Introduction to the case

This case shows a patient with recurrent VTs after MI. LV endocardial mapping in sinus rhythm revealed the following electrograms (Figure 49.1).

Figure 49.1 Electrogram recordings of the LV endocardium in sinus rhythm. Map: proximal, distal, and unipolar signal from the mapping catheter

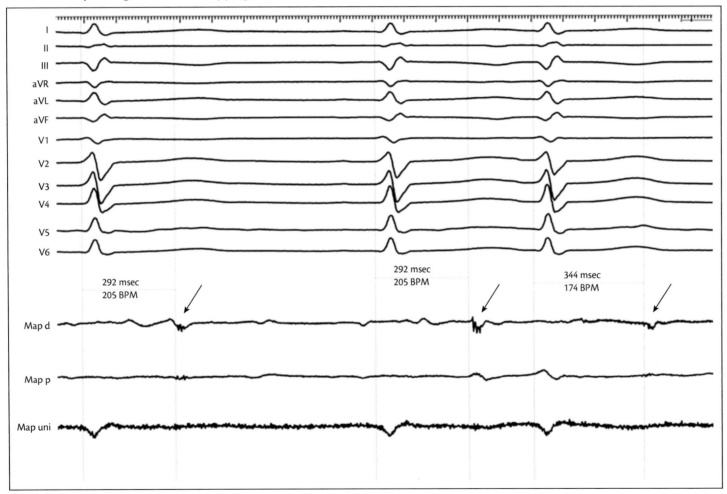

Question

Electrograms annotated by arrows are:

A   Artefacts—due to absence of fixed relation to the QRS complex

B   Atrial potentials

C   Electrograms from the conduction system

D   Late potentials within the dense scar region

E   Late potentials at the periphery of the scar

Answer

D Late potentials within the dense scar region

Explanation

Late potentials with decremental conduction in post-myocardial infarction scar

The electrograms represent late potentials recorded over the narrow channel of slow conduction within the dense post-infarction scar (only far-field ventricular electrograms corresponding to the QRS complex are recorded). Note the decremental conduction within the channel that manifests after a premature atrial beat (3rd complex of the recording).

When isoprenaline was administered, the coupling interval of the late potential shortened to 155ms and slow VT could be induced.

Catheter ablation focused on elimination of all late potentials could be one of the endpoints of an ablation procedure for VT in structural heart disease.[1–5]

References

1. Aliot EM, Stevenson WG, Almendral-Garrote JM *et al*. EHRA/HRS expert consensus on catheter ablation of ventricular arrhythmias. *Heart Rhythm* 2009; **6**: 886–933.

2. Jaïs P, Maury P, Khairy P, *et al*. Elimination of local abnormal ventricular activities: a new end point for substrate modification in patients with scar-related ventricular tachycardia. *Circulation* 2012; **125**: 2184–96.

3. Tilz RR, Makimoto H, Rillig A, *et al*. Electrical isolation of a substrate after myocardial infarction: a novel ablation strategy for unmappable ventricular tachycardias—feasibility and clinical outcome. *Europace* 2014; **16**: 1040–52.

4. Mountantonakis SE, Park RE, Frankel DS, *et al*. Relationship between voltage map 'channels' and the location of critical isthmus sites in patients with post-infarction cardiomyopathy and ventricular tachycardia. *J Am Coll Cardiol* 2013; **61**: 2088–95.

5. Vergara P, Trevisi N, Ricco A, *et al*. Late potentials abolition as an additional technique for reduction of arrhythmia recurrence in scar related ventricular tachycardia ablation. *J Cardiovasc Electrophysiol* 2012; **23**: 621–7.

Introduction to the case

Fractionated electrograms are frequently recorded in infarcted myocardium and are caused by asynchronous activation in areas where myocardial and collagen fibres intermingle (Figure 50.1). Selection of the activation time in a unipolar fractionated electrogram is a challenge.

Figure 50.1 Depiction of a fractionated unipolar electrogram. stim: stimulation artefact; ms: milliseconds

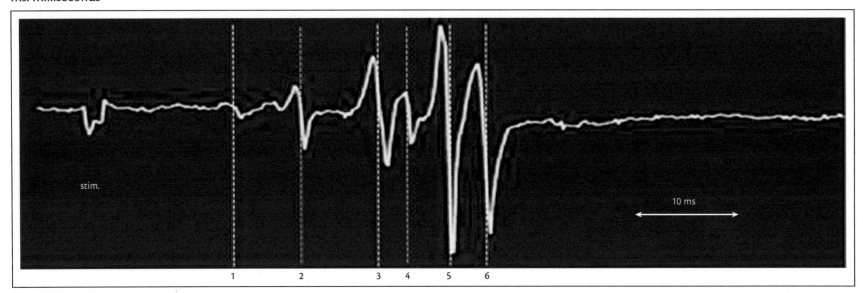

Question

The local activation time in the fractionated electrogram shown is:

A The 1st deflection (1)

B The deflection with the steepest negative dV/dt (5)

C The 4th deflection

D The last deflection (6)

E Impossible to define

Answer

E **Impossible to define**

Explanation

Fractionated electrograms

It is impossible to determine the activation time in a fractionated electrogram from a single recording.[1-4] The tracings (Figure 50.2) show the original tracing (tracing b) together with a recording made at a site 1mm above (tracing a) and 1mm below (tracing c) the recording site of tracing b. The deflection marked with the white dot in tracing b has corresponding deflections (occurring at exactly the same time) in tracings a and c. These are, however, lower in amplitude in tracings a and c, indicating that they are remote and caused by the activation running underneath electrode b. The same applies for the deflection in tracing b marked by the blue dot, indicating that this deflection too is a local one. All other deflections in tracing b have similar deflections in the two neighbouring tracings, but the amplitude in tracing b is always lower than the corresponding deflection in tracing a or c, indicating that these

deflections of tracing b are remote. Thus, in this example, there are two local deflections (4 and 5) in tracing b.

References

1. Anderson KP, Walker R, Ershler PR, *et al*. Determination of local myocardial electrical activation for activation sequence mapping: a statistical approach. *Circ Res* 1991; **69**: 898–917.

2. de Bakker JMT, Hauer RNW, Simmers TA (1995). Activation mapping: unipolar versus bipolar recording. In: DP Zipes, J Jalife (eds.). *Cardiac Electrophysiology: From Cell to Bedside*, 2nd edn. Philadelphia: WB Saunders Company, pp. 1068–78.

3. de Bakker JM, Wittkampf FH. The pathophysiologic basis of fractionated and complex electrograms and the impact of recording techniques on their detection and interpretation. *Circ Arrhythm Electrophysiol* 2010; **3**: 204–13.

4. Jacquemet V, Henriquez CS. Genesis of complex fractionated atrial electrograms in zones of slow conduction: a computer model of microfibrosis. *Heart Rhythm* 2009; **6**: 803–10.

Figure 50.2 The original tracing (Figure 50.1) together with a recording made at a site 1mm above and 1mm below the recording site of the original tracing

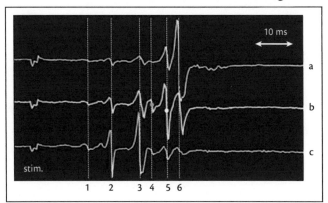

Introduction to the case

This case presents a 61-year-old woman with ischaemic cardiomyopathy and palpitations (Figure 51.1).

During an electrophysiological study (Figure 51.2), clinical narrow complex tachycardia was induced.

Figure 51.1 (a) Spontaneous narrow complex (104ms), 'irregular' tachycardia. (b) Sinus rhythm

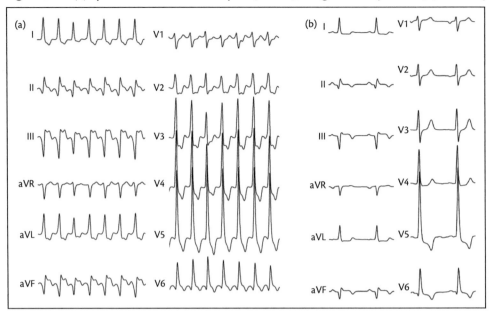

Figure 51.2 Surface leads II and V3 and intracardiac recordings from the high right atrium (HRA), His bundle (HB), coronary sinus (CS), and right ventricular apex (RVA)

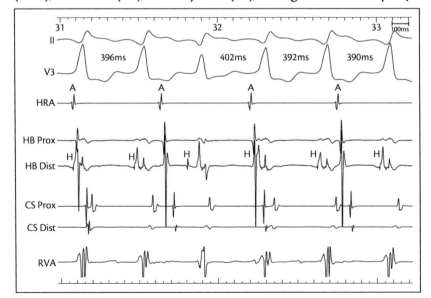

Question

The mechanism of tachycardia is:

A VT from the proximal His–Purkinje system

B BBRVT

C AVNRT or junctional ectopic tachycardia

D Orthodromic AVRT via nodo-fascicular pathway

E Pre-excited tachycardia

Answer

A VT from the proximal His–Purkinje system

Explanation

Ventricular tachycardia from the proximal His–Purkinje system

This patient presented with a tachycardia with borderline QRS width. The narrower QRS complex (3rd beat) is the result of a sinus impulse with His bundle (HB) capture. The salient features of this tachycardia are: (1) the relatively narrow QRS complex configuration (near-identical to sinus rhythm); (2) VA dissociation with capture beats; and (3) the positive, but short, local HV interval. The differential diagnosis of narrow complex tachycardia with VA dissociation includes junctional ectopic tachycardia (JET), AVNRT with block in the upper common pathway, orthodromic nodo-fascicular (NF)/nodo-ventricular (NV) re-entry, and a focal tachycardia from the proximal or distal His–Purkinje system. JET, based upon abnormal automaticity originating above the bifurcation of the HB, is normally seen in children, and VA conduction can be observed transiently in the majority of cases. Moreover, during JET originating above the HB, the HV interval is expected to be similar to that during sinus rhythm. AVNRT with block to the atria and orthodromic re-entry involving a NF/NV pathway (both rare) are ruled out by the shortening of the HV interval during tachycardia. Most likely, this narrow complex tachycardia with VA dissociation and short local HV interval can be explained by a focal tachycardia from the proximal His–Purkinje system. Because of the infra-Hisian origin, VA dissociation can occur without interrupting the tachycardia. The short local HV interval is only a reflection of the shorter time it takes the focus to get retrogradely to the HB versus its exit site to the ventricle. The relative narrowness of the QRS complexes (and near-identical morphology as during sinus rhythm) is explained by its origin in (or exit close to) the proximal His–Purkinje network (proximal left bundle). The capture cycles also favour the involvement of the normal conduction system in the tachycardia mechanism.

Note: proof that the initial sharp deflection indicated by 'H' really is a His potential is given by the absence of this potential during the captured complex (the negative component can easily be seen to be absent).

Introduction to the case

Case 12 introduces a 14-year-old boy with no structural heart disease but recurrent episodes of wide complex, AV synchronous tachycardia (390ms). Because of the incessant nature, catheters were placed during tachycardia. No clear His was recorded (Figure 52.1a). Atrial overdrive pacing (320ms) was performed, after which the tachycardia continued (Figure 52.1b).

Figure 52.1 (a) No clear His was recorded. (b) Atrial overdrive pacing. Surface leads II, V1, and V6 and intracardiac recordings from the high right atrium (HRA), His bundle (HB), coronary sinus (CS), and right ventricular apex (RVA)

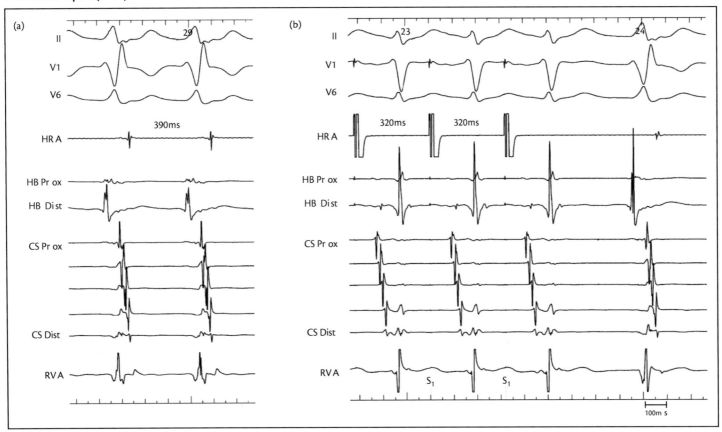

Question

In this adolescent, the mechanism of tachycardia is:

A   AT with right bundle branch aberrancy

B   Fascicular left VT

C   AVNRT with right bundle branch aberrancy

D   Antidromic AVRT

E   BBRVT

Answer

B   Fascicular left VT

Explanation

Fascicular ventricular tachycardia

This patient presented with an incessant tachycardia with a right bundle branch block morphology. No His deflection was recorded despite a correct fluoroscopic position. There was a 1-to-1 relation between the atrium and ventricle with the earliest A (small deflection) at the His catheter. Together with the young age of the patient, the finding of an AV synchronous tachycardia may suggest AVNRT (or AT) with right bundle branch aberrancy. During atrial overdrive pacing (Figure 52.1b), there was acceleration of the ventricle, with normalization of the QRS morphology and appearance of a distinct His before the local ventricular deflection. After cessation of pacing, tachycardia continued with a long PPI interval and an 'AVVA' response. The above pacing manoeuvre is indicative for VT and is explained by a continuous reset of the VT by atrial overdrive pacing (equivalent of constant capture beats). In fact, the 'AVVA' response is the reciprocal image of a 'VAAV' response observed after overdrive pacing of atrial tachycardia. There is no evidence of fusion (entrainment). The diagnosis of VT explains the disappearance of a His deflection during tachycardia (i.e. masked within the V deflection during retrograde conduction from the focus, over the node to the atrium). The absence of a His deflection cannot be explained by AVNRT, AT, orthodromic AVRT, or BBRVT in which a clear His is expected to precede the local V. Only during antidromic AVRT can a His get buried into the ventricular deflection (during retrograde His bundle activation). This case, however, is not an antidromic AVRT (not a pre-excited QRS, normalization of the QRS during atrial overdrive pacing, AVVA response, etc.).

The final diagnosis was fascicular left VT with 1-to-1 VA conduction. During adenosine challenge, the tachycardia continued with a VA block. This case illustrates the diagnostic utility of atrial pacing manoeuvres during wide complex tachycardia.

Introduction to the case

Case 53 refers to a 25-year-old teacher with palpitations and who has intermittent LBBB on ECG recordings. He develops the following tachycardia at an electrophysiological study. During sinus rhythm without bundle branch block, a clear His electrogram was visible but always 'disappeared' during tachycardia since it coincided with the local ventricular electrograms. A diagnostic manoeuvre (Figure 53.1) is performed with a PAC delivered from the high right atrium.

Figure 53.1 Surface leads II, aVF, V1, and V6 and intracardiac recordings from the high right atrium (HRA), the proximal, mid, and distal bipoles of the His bundle (His), the proximal to distal bipoles of the coronary sinus (CS), and the right ventricular apex (RVA).

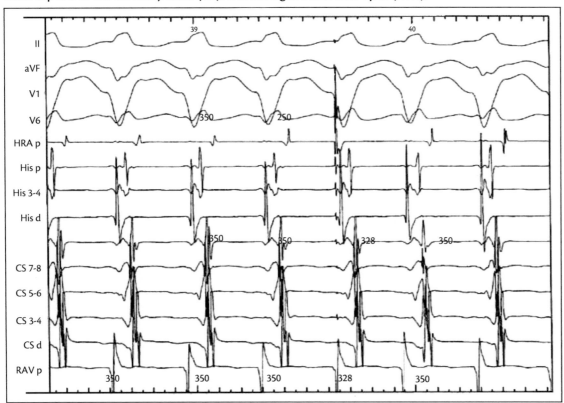

Question

The tracing demonstrates:

A   An AT with bundle branch block

B   Termination of the tachycardia and re-initiation of a 2nd tachycardia

C   BBRVT

D   Resetting of an atrio-fascicular AVRT

E   Resetting of AVNRT

Answer

D   Resetting of an atrio-fascicular AVRT

Explanation

An atrial extrastimulus during wide complex tachycardia

The surface ECG demonstrates an LBBB tachycardia with no clear His electrogram despite its presence in sinus rhythm. The differential is that of VT or an antidromic AVRT. The left bundle pattern looks like a typical LBBB, and the RV apex activates before the onset of the surface QRS and the His bundle ventricular electrogram. The premature atrial beat delivered during AV nodal refractoriness advances the RV apical electrogram and resets the tachycardia with advancement of the next atrial electrogram (CS prox), with the same retrograde activation sequence. This resetting of the tachycardia circuit by a premature atrial beat, with the RV apex preceding surface ECG QRS and His ventricular electrogram, is a diagnostic feature of an atrio-fascicular pathway (Mahaim pathway).[1] For atrial tachycardia and AVNRT, the His bundle deflection had to come in front of the ventricular electrogram and QRS. Also for BBRVT, the His bundle should precede the QRS. It is not possible that a 2nd tachycardia has been initiated as there is no change in the surface ECG or activation sequence on the intracardiac electrograms.

References

1. Tchou P, Lehman MH, Jazayeri M, *et al* Atriofascicular connection or a nodoventricular Mahaim fiber? Electrophysiological elucidation of the pathway and associated reentrant circuit. *Circulation* 1988; **77**: 837–48.

Introduction to the case

Case 54 involves a patient after previous MI with tolerated VT. During programmed ventricular stimulation, clinical VT with a cycle length of 510ms was induced. LV mapping within the scar region revealed discrete diastolic potentials. At this site, pacing was performed (at rate of 30ms shorter than TCL) (Figure 54.1).

Figure 54.1 Entrainment manoeuvre from the LV endocardium during VT. Abl: mapping catheter; RVA: right ventricular apex

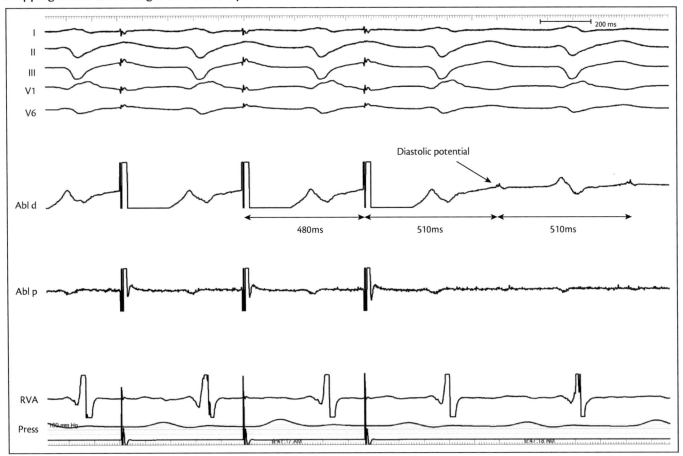

Question

What is the correct statement?

A   The manoeuvre shows entrainment with fusion

B   The catheter is positioned within the outer loop of the re-entrant circuit

C   The catheter is positioned in the remote bystander region

D   The catheter is positioned within the exit zone of slow conduction

E   Termination of arrhythmia by ablation at this site is likely

Answer

E   **Termination of arrhythmia by ablation at this site is likely**

Explanation

Entrainment with concealed fusion of a ventricular tachycardia

VT is entrained without change of QRS morphology which is called entrainment with concealed fusion. Entrainment with fusion (i.e. change of QRS morphology) is typical for outer loop and/or remote bystander region.

The PPI matches the cycle length of the tachycardia which confirms active participation of the site in the re-entrant circuit.

The catheter is located inside the central zone of slow conduction since S–QRS is within 31–50% of the VT cycle length. For the exit site, the S–QRS interval should be <30% of the VT cycle length.[1-3]

Pacing manoeuvre identifies the protected isthmus of slow conduction of the re-entrant circuit and ablation at this site is very likely to terminate the arrhythmia.

References

1. Stevenson WG, Sager PT, Friedman PL. Entrainment techniques for mapping atrial and ventricular tachycardias. *J Cardiovasc Electrophysiol* 1995; **6**: 201–16.

2. Waldo AL. From bedside to bench: entrainment and other stories. *Heart Rhythm* 2004; **1**: 94–106.

3. Stevenson WG, Friedman PL, Sager PT,*et al.* Exploring postinfarction reentrant ventricular tachycardia with entrainment mapping. *J Am Coll Cardiol* 1997; **29**: 1180–9.

Introduction to the case

The patient in Case 55 shows recurrent post-MI VT and documented aneurysm of the LV inferior wall filled with an old organized thrombus. Endocardial activation mapping revealed no mid-diastolic activity either in the LV or RV (only signals corresponding with entrance or exit sites on both sides of the thrombus). The depicted electrogram (Figure 55.1) was recorded within the proximal CS.

Figure 55.1 (a) Intracardiac echocardiogram depicting an old organized thrombus (arrows) in the LV aneurysm. (b) LV electroanatomical voltage map (LV inferior view) showing scar region with superimposed thrombus (grey area). (c) Intracardiac recordings during VT (proximal CS)

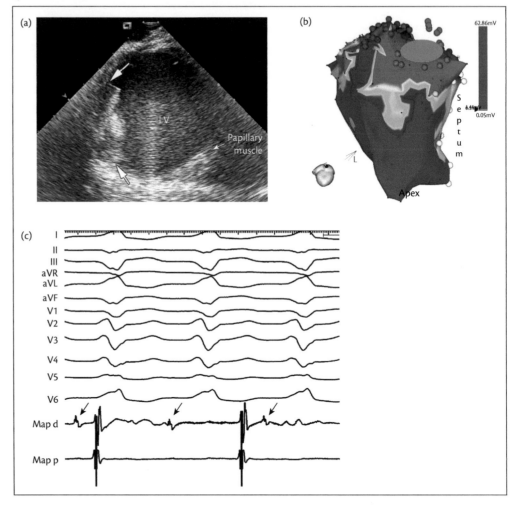

Question

The signals marked by arrows represent:

A Atrial potentials within the CS

B Electrograms originating in the conduction system

C Mid-diastolic potentials suggestive of critical zone of slow conduction of re-entrant circuit (protected isthmus)

D Far-field electrograms from the LV endocardium

E Electrograms corresponding to entrance zone of slow conduction of re-entrant circuit

Answer

C Mid-diastolic potentials suggestive of critical zone of slow conduction of re-entrant circuit (protected isthmus)

Explanation

Mid-diastolic potentials during ventricular tachycardia recorded from the coronary sinus

The timing of the local electrogram corresponds to the central zone of the re-entrant circuit that could be epicardial in patients after an inferior wall MI. Pacing at this site showed concealed entrainment. Catheter ablation terminated VT within a few seconds. The presence of a thrombus did not affect the result of catheter ablation. Mapping in the CS and/or venous tributaries should be considered before epicardial access.[1–4]

References

1. Kautzner J, Bytesník J, Cihák R, Vancura V. Radiofrequency catheter ablation of postinfarction ventricular tachycardia from the proximal coronary sinus. *J Cardiovasc Electrophysiol* 2001; **12**: 363–6.

2. Doppalapudi H, Yamada T, Ramaswamy K, *et al*. Idiopathic focal epicardial ventricular tachycardia originating from the crux of the heart. *Heart Rhythm* 2009; **6**: 44–50.

3. Baher A, Shah DJ, Valderrabano M. Coronary venous ethanol infusion for the treatment of refractory ventricular tachycardia. *Heart Rhythm* 2012; **9**: 1637–9.

4. Reithmann C, Fiek M, Hahnefeld A, *et al*. Recording of low-amplitude diastolic electrograms through the coronary veins: a guide for epicardial ventricular tachycardia ablation. *Europace* 2012; **14**: 865–71.

Introduction to the case

A 15-year-old male presenting for follow-up is discussed in this case. This surface ECG (Figure 56.1) was recorded 1 year following the ablation of a posteroseptal accessory pathway. Because of his ECG, a new EP study was planned.

The tracings in Figure 56.2 were recorded during incremental atrial pacing.

Figure 56.1 Surface ECG. 25mm/s, 10mm/mV

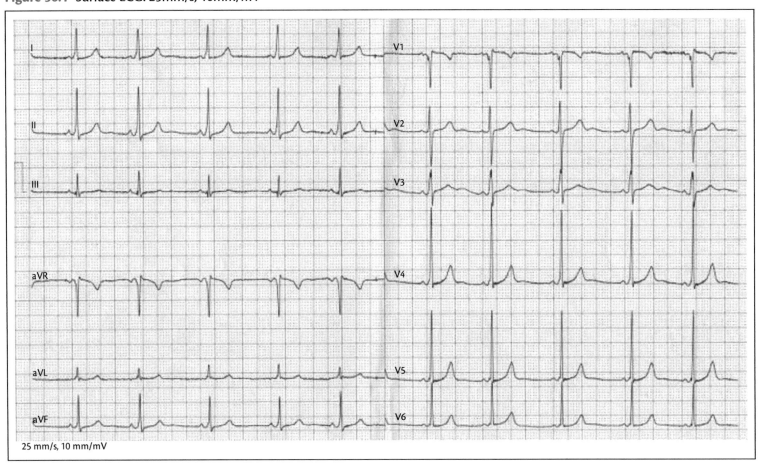

25 mm/s, 10 mm/mV

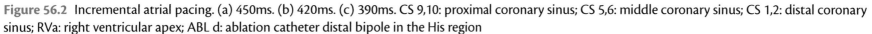

Figure 56.2 Incremental atrial pacing. (a) 450ms. (b) 420ms. (c) 390ms. CS 9,10: proximal coronary sinus; CS 5,6: middle coronary sinus; CS 1,2: distal coronary sinus; RVa: right ventricular apex; ABL d: ablation catheter distal bipole in the His region

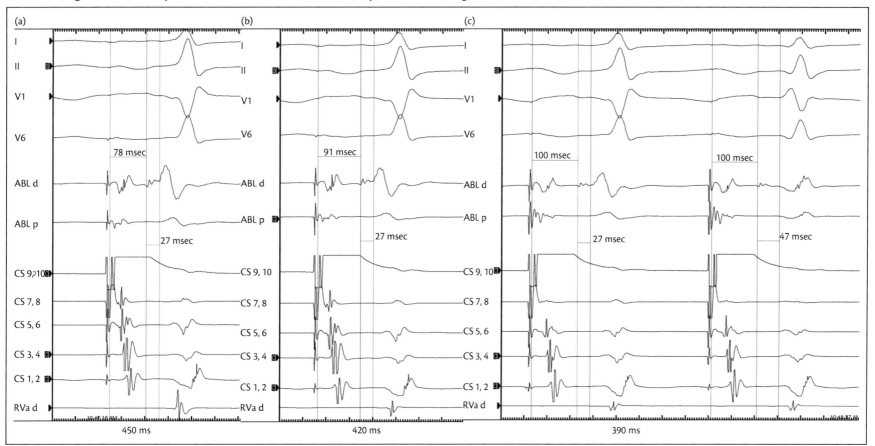

Question

Which is the best explanation for this finding?

A The posteroseptal accessory pathway recurred

B There is a 2nd AV accessory pathway and the ablation should be performed in the para-His region

C There is no need for ablation because this pathway is not capable of sustaining tachycardia

D There is no pre-excitation

E Dual AV nodal pathways

Answer

C **There is no need for ablation because this pathway is not capable of sustaining tachycardia**

Explanation

Looking at pre-excitation

During atrial pacing at progressively shorter cycle lengths, the AH interval prolonged and the HV interval remained the same at 27ms. Also the QRS configuration during atrial pacing at increasing rates remained unaltered. At 390ms, there is block in the pathway with conduction through the AV node with a normal HV interval of 47ms on the last tracing. All these findings support a fasciculo-ventricular pathway. Fasciculo-ventricular pathways are rare variants of ventricular pre-excitation. They take off from the His bundle or bundle branch and insert into the ventricular septum, are not capable of sustaining re-entry, and do not participate in re-entrant circuits. They are considered an ECG curiosity.[1] It is important to identify a fasciculo-ventricular pathway and avoid ablation because of possible damage to the AV node.[2, 3]

References

1. Josephson ME (2002). *Clinical Cardiac Electrophysiology: Techniques and Interpretations*, 3rd edn. Philadelphia: Lippincott, Williams, & Wilkins.

2. Sternick EB, Gerken LM, Vrandecic MO, Wellens HJJ. Fasciculoventricular pathways: clinical and electrophysiologic characteristics of a variant of preexcitation. *J Cardiovasc Electrophysiol* 2003; **14**: 1057–63.

3. Sternick EB, Oliva A, Wellens HJJ, *et al*. Clinical, electrocardiographic, and electrophysiologic characteristics of patients with a fasciculoventricular pathway: the role of PRKAG2 mutation. *Heart Rhythm* 2011; **8**: 58–64.

Introduction to the case

This case discusses a PVC tracing. Figure 57.1 displays this.

Figure 57.1 PVC tracing

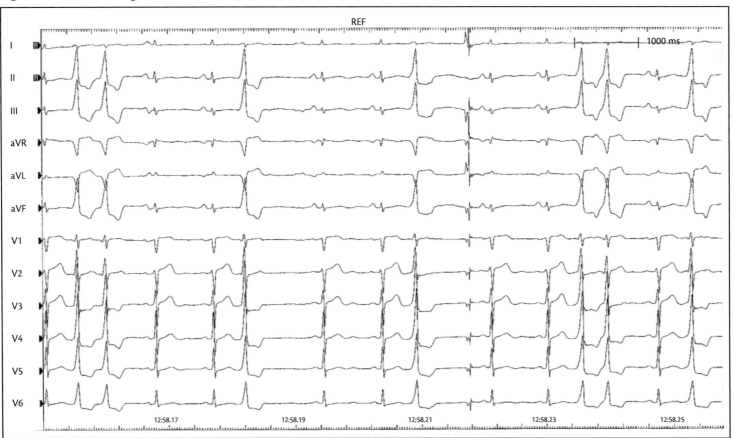

Question

What is the origin of the PVC? The correct diagnosis is:

A   Right ventricular outflow tract (RVOT)

B   Aortic cusps or left ventricular outflow tract (LVOT)

C   Aortic–mitral continuity

D   Epicardial perivascular (distal CS)

E   Aortic cusps or LVOT or epicardial perivascular (distal CS, AIV)

Answer

E   Aortic cusps or LVOT or epicardial perivascular (distal CS)

Explanation

Where do these VPBs come from?

The positive R wave on V1 and V2–3 rules out the RVOT as the origin of the PVC (Figure 57.2 and Figure 57.3). The mitral valve is also not possible, because V1 is not entirely positive. This PVC could originate from the aortic cusps, LVOT, or epicardium. This case was found slightly below the cusp (Figure 57.4). Often, despite the presence of good algorithms in literature, it is better to anticipate mapping in the RV, LV, aorta, and CS in most of outflow tract cases (Figure 57.5).

Figure 57.2 PVC

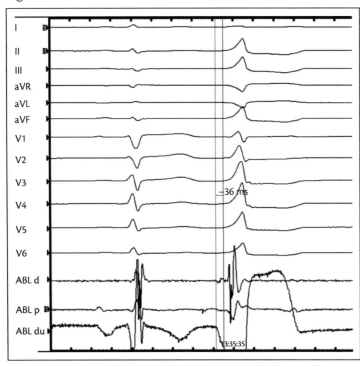

Figure 57.3 PVC

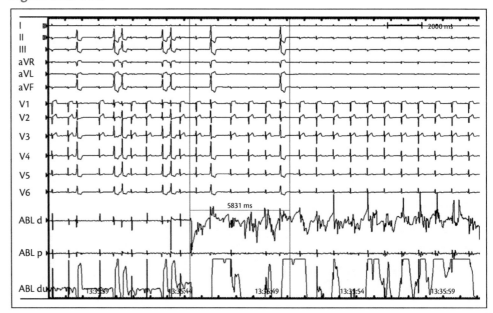

Figure 57.4 (a) Right anterior oblique

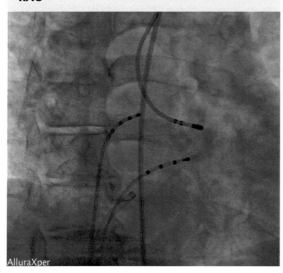

Figure 57.4 (b) Left anterior oblique

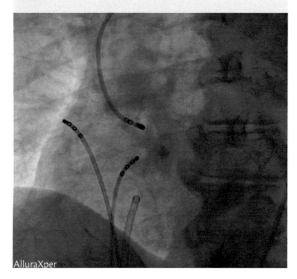

Figure 57.5 Surface lead recordings during sinus rhythm and monomorphic premature ventricular contractions (PVC). Niloufar Tabatabaei and Samuel J. Asirvatham, Supravalvular Arrhythmia: Identifying and Ablating the Substrate; *Circulation: Arrhythmia and Electrophysiology* Vol. 2, No. 3, 2009 with permission from Wolters Kluwer.

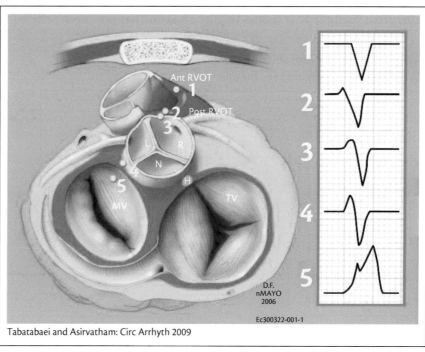

Introduction to the case

A 24-year-old woman with recurrent ventricular fibrillation (VF) is presented in Case 58. The patient had been resuscitated after a sudden cardiac arrest 3 years ago. There was no underlying structural heart disease present and she was implanted with an ICD. She did suffer from multiple ICD shocks (Figure 58.1) and has now been referred for VF ablation.

Figure 58.1 Abl d: distal ablation catheter; His d: distal His bundle; His p: proximal His bundle

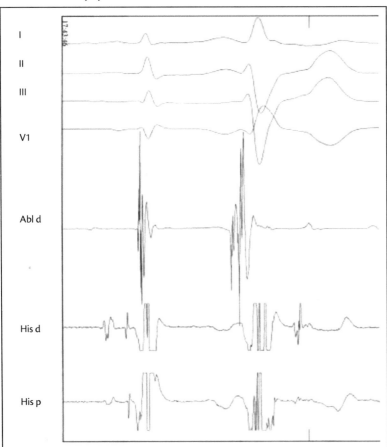

Question

Where does the 2nd beat come from?

A Right bundle branch

B CS

C Left Purkinje network

D Left lateral ventricle close to the mitral annulus

E LVOT

Answer

C   **Left Purkinje network**

Explanation

Looking closely at ventricular premature beats

The 1st beat is a sinus beat. The ablation catheter (Abl dist) displays a sharp potential (Figure 58.2) (Purkinje potential, shown by the arrow)[1] of <15ms before the ventricular electrogram. During the PVC, the sharp potential becomes earlier and is situated before QRS onset. Typically seen in left Purkinje PVC, the QRS is pretty narrow. Targeting PVC initiating VF may suppress VF episodes.[2]

References

1. Haïssaguerre M, Shah DC, Jaïs P, *et al.* Role of Purkinje conducting system in triggering of idiopathic ventricular fibrillation. *Lancet* 2002; **359**: 677–8.

2. Haïssaguerre M, Shoda M, Jaïs P, *et al.* Mapping and ablation of idiopathic ventricular fibrillation. *Circulation* 2002; **106**: 962–7.

Figure 58.2 Purkinje potential

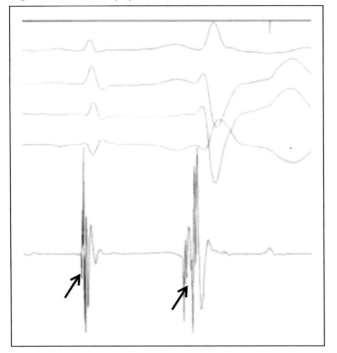

Introduction to the case

A 67-year-old man referred for VT ablation is discussed in this case. This patient had an inferior MI 10 years ago. No revascularization was attempted at that time. His LVEF is now 30%. Because of recurrent ICD therapies despite beta-blockers and amiodarone, he was referred for VT ablation. Ventricular TCL was 520ms; pacing was at 450ms from the tip of the ablation catheter (Figure 59.1).

Figure 59.1 Electrophysiological study during entrainment manoeuvres. RFd: distal bipole of the ablation catheter; RFp: proximal bipole of the ablation catheter; RV 1-2: distal bipole of the catheter placed at the RV apex; CS 1-2: distal bipole of the catheter placed in the coronary sinus; S: stimulation

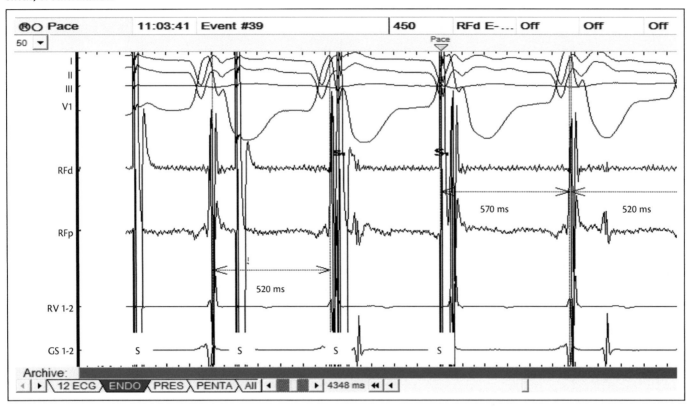

Question

Which part of the VT circuit is paced?

A Not possible to say as there is no capture

B At the exit of the VT isthmus

C In an outer loop

D At the entrance of the VT isthmus

E In a bystander area

Answer

A Not possible to say as there is no capture

Explanation

Interpreting entrainment during ventricular tachycardia

The TCL remains at 520ms during pacing despite a pacing interval at 450ms. There is no ventricular capture or entrainment of the tachycardia, and the measured return cycle of 570ms after the last pacing cycle is meaningless. Therefore, there is no usable information and entrainment should be redone.[1,2]

References

1. Stevenson WG, Khan H, Sager P, *et al*. Identification of reentry circuit sites during catheter mapping and radiofrequency ablation of ventricular tachycardia late after myocardial infarction. *Circulation* 1993; **88**: 1647–70.

2. Stevenson WG, Friedman PL, Sager PT, *et al*. Exploring postinfarction reentrant ventricular tachycardia with entrainment mapping. *J Am Coll Cardiol* 1997; **29**: 1180–9.

Introduction to the case

Case 60 discusses a patient after an anterior and inferior MI, a coronary artery bypass graft, and a cardiac arrest, and with recurrent VTs in the ICD memory. LV endocardial mapping during arrhythmia (cycle length 420ms) revealed an entrance zone in the low septum with concealed entrainment. Ablation at this site terminated VT. However, the following VT (Figure 60.1) was induced after ablation with these electrograms higher at the septum.

Figure 60.1 Ventricular tachycardia. Abl: proximal, distal, and unipolar signal from the mapping catheter; RVA: catheter in RV apex

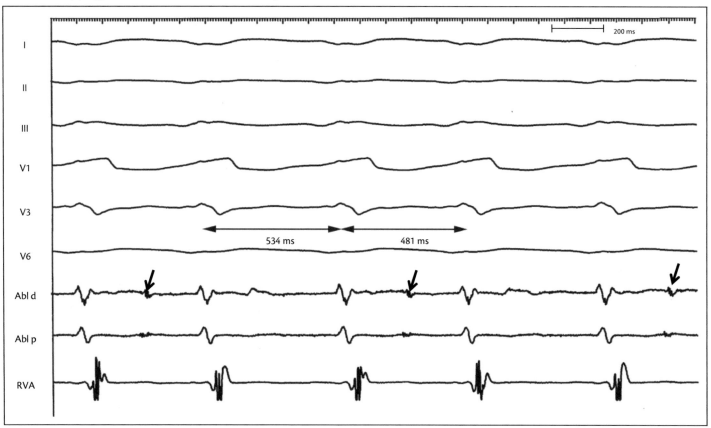

Question

Electrograms annotated by arrows are most likely:

A Artefacts due to its inconsistent appearance

B Far-field atrial signals during 2:1 VA conduction

C Mid-diastolic potentials that do not participate in documented VT due to 2:1 conduction

D Electrograms originating in the conduction system (late activation)

E Mid-diastolic potentials suggesting the presence of two channels of slow conduction with one common exit site

239

Answer

E **Mid-diastolic potentials suggesting the presence of two channels of slow conduction with one common exit site**

Explanation

Ventricular tachycardia with alternating cycle lengths

After ablation within the entrance zone in the low septum, VT has alternating cycle lengths with two different rates, but the same QRS morphology. This suggests the presence of two separate protected channels with different conduction properties, but with a common exit site.[1-3]

The mid-diastolic potentials recorded higher on the septum are present only for one VT cycle length and reflect the activation of one channel of slow conduction.

The catheter was moved even higher at the septum and mid-diastolic signals were present at a 1:1 ratio (i.e. closer to the exit site). Pacing manoeuvres were difficult to apply due to alternating cycle lengths. Catheter ablation terminated the VT.

References

1. Stevenson WG, Sager PT, Friedman PL. Entrainment techniques for mapping atrial and ventricular tachycardias. *J Cardiovasc Electrophysiol* 1995; **6**: 201–16.

2. Waldo AL. From bedside to bench: entrainment and other stories. *Heart Rhythm* 2004; **1**: 94–106.

3. Stevenson WG, Friedman PL, Sager PT *et al.* Exploring postinfarction reentrant ventricular tachycardia with entrainment mapping. *J Am Coll Cardiol* 1997; **29**: 1180–9.

Introduction to the case

This case presents a man of 69 years with bronchial asthma and his evaluation of the RSPV at the end of ipsilateral vein encircling (pacing at the proximal CS is switched on and off) (Figure 61.1).

Figure 61.1 (a) Sinus rhythm. (b) Pacing at CSp. (c) Sinus rhythm. (d) Pacing at CSp

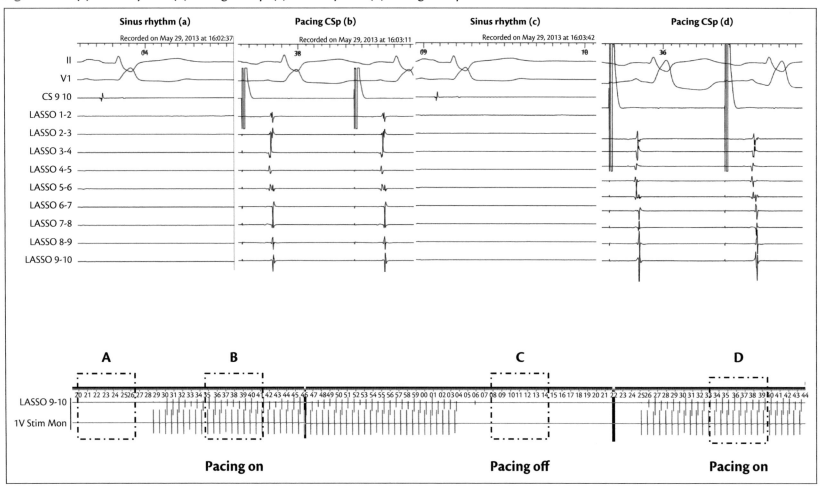

Question

The tracings show:

A The RSPV is characterized by exit block

B The RSPV is not isolated (no entry block) and additional ablation is required

C The RSPV is definitely isolated (entry block both during sinus rhythm and pacing at CSp)

D The right inferior pulmonary vein (RIPV) is not isolated

E A and C

Answer

B **The RSPV is not isolated (no entry block) and additional ablation is required**

Explanation

Dormant conduction requiring additional ablation

At first glance, isolation was observed, as evidenced by the absence of PV potentials during sinus rhythm (cycle length of 1320ms) (Figure 61.1a). Interestingly however, immediately thereafter pacing at CSp (cycle length of 700ms) unmasked residual entry conduction into the RSPV, as evidenced by delayed PV potentials at Lasso (Figure 61.1b). Dormant PV conduction was reconfirmed by 'switching off (Figure 61.1c) and on' (Figure 61.1d) pacing at the CSp, proving that the observation was not just a time-dependent reconnection.

Additional ablation at the gap in the anterior part of the circle (not shown) completely eliminated entry conduction into the RSPV, as evidenced by the disappearance of PV potentials at Lasso during pacing at the CSp. The underlying mechanism is unproven, but it is likely to be caused by ablation-induced anisotropy at the 'gap'. Therefore, one may observe residual (but delayed) conduction into the PV during CSp pacing (uniform and linear wavefront), without conduction (entrance block) during sinus rhythm (curved and elliptical wavefront).

Note: the alternative hypothesis of intra-atrial block (i.e. region of CS and veins isolated from the rest of the left atrium) is unlikely, given the presence of CS potentials during sinus rhythm.

Introduction to the case

During an electrophysiological study in a woman aged 17, SVT was induced by programmed stimulation. The onset of one of the episodes of tachycardia is shown (Figure 62.1).

Figure 62.1 First beats of an episode of SVT, induced by rapid atrial pacing. RAA: right atrial appendage; HBp till HBd: His bundle recordings from proximal to distal; PS: posteroseptal recording; CS: coronary sinus; A: atrial electrogram; H: His bundle deflection; S: stimulus

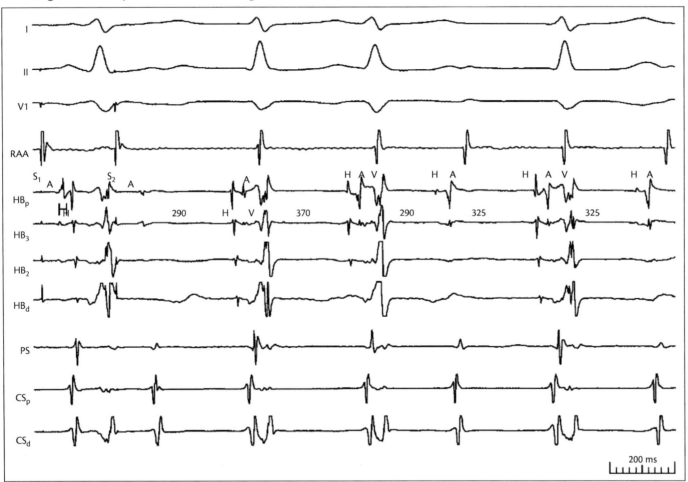

Question

What describes the tracing best?

A AT is induced

B AVRT with (nodal) Wenckebach block

C AVRT with infra-nodal block

D Slow/fast AVNRT with (nodal) Wenckebach block

E Slow/fast AVNRT with infra-nodal block

Answer

E Slow/fast AVNRT with infra-nodal block

Explanation

2:1 block during supraventricular tachycardia

An atrial extrastimulus (S_2) during right atrial pacing (S_1) at a cycle length of 600ms induces an SVT with an irregular cycle length and variable AV conduction (A > V). AVRT is excluded because of the AV dissociation. The mode of initiation, the atrial activation sequence, and the fact that A–A oscillations follow, rather than precede, H–H oscillations are all arguments against an AT.

The earliest atrial activation at the anterior septum is compatible with slow/fast AVNRT. Oscillations in the A–H interval with a long–short sequence lead to A–V block in the beat with a shorter H–H interval (290ms) after a longer H–H interval (370ms; beat three of the tachycardia). A proximal abortive His bundle (*H*) potential is recorded in the blocked complexes, while activation along the full right bundle branch can be seen in the conducted beats.

Although the H–H interval before the last beat of the tachycardia is similar to the last but one, infra-His block occurs due to the long–short sequence as a result of the preceding blocked beat. Once initiated, such 2:1 block can continue for a long time due to the persistent long–short alternation, resulting in long Purkinje system refractoriness after long H–H intervals.

Since typical slow/fast AVNRT has no LCP, if 2:1 AV block during tachycardia is present, it is always infra-nodal in nature.[1] The abortive proximal His bundle electrograms can be much smaller than in this example but can always be found. In contrast, atypical AVNRT which has an LCP can show 2:1 AV conduction due to low nodal block.

References

1. Heidbuchel H, Jackman WM. Characterization of subforms of AV nodal reentrant tachycardia. *Europace* 2004; **6**: 316–29.

Introduction to the case

A woman, aged 33, with paroxysmal SVT is referred for ablation. Typical slow/fast AVNRT is diagnosed and characterized during an electrophysiological study. Figure 63.1 shows the position of the catheters inside the heart during the diagnostic study, both in the RAO and LAO projections. The figure also shows five locations to choose from in order to ablate the slow AV nodal pathway.

Figure 63.1 (a) RAO. (b) LAO. RAA: right atrial appendage; HB: His bundle; CS: coronary sinus; Map: mapping catheter; RAO: right anterior oblique; LAO: left anterior oblique. The blue circle denotes the ostium of the coronary sinus.

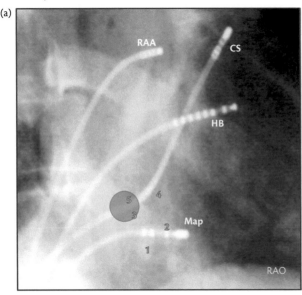 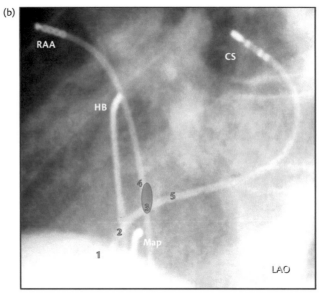

Question

Regardless of electrograms, which anatomical site is the best one to start ablation, since it is most likely to induce junctional rhythm and ablate antegrade slow pathway conduction, with the lowest risk to harm the fast AV nodal pathway?

A   Site 1

B   Site 2

C   Site 3

D   Site 4

E   Site 5

Answer

B   Site 2

Explanation

The radiological anatomy of slow pathway ablation

The connection of the slow AV pathway and the atrium runs alongside the tricuspid annulus, in between the tricuspid annulus and the CS ostium (Figure 63.2). Although it is often believed that the anterior edge of the CS ostium (location 3 in Figure 63.1) is the location where the slow pathway can best be targeted, more recent data from three-dimensional right atrial visualization and overlay with fluoroscopy have indicated that the part of the atrium just inside the tricuspid annulus is the location

where a junctional rhythm is most often induced with successful ensuing slow pathway ablation (location 2; see also Figure 63.2 in another patient, in which the pink dot was the site of junctional rhythm induction and successful ablation).[1,2]

Starting too far away from the septum (location 1) makes no sense since this will not be able to interrupt the slow pathway conduction. Although applications inside the CS (location 5) may sometimes be required (in

Figure 63.2 Overlay of the three-dimensional anatomy of the right atrium with real-time fluoroscopy made with LARCA software, after three-dimensional rotational angiography on a syngo DynaCT (Siemens AG, Erlangen, Germany)

Reproduced from Stijn De Buck *et al*, Asymmetric collimation can significantly reduce patient radiation dose during pulmonary vein isolation, *Europace*, Vol. 14, No. 3 (2012) with permission from Oxford University Press

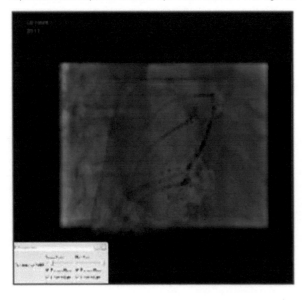
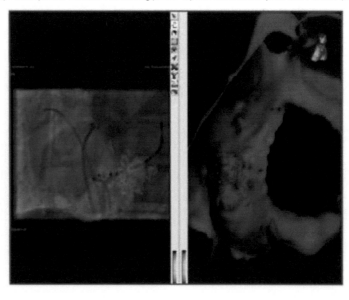

case of a so-called left-sided variant of AVNRT), this occurs only in <2% of AVNRT. In some patients, applications higher on the septum, at the level of the upper margin of the CS ostium (location 4 in Figure 63.1) are needed for success, but this location is associated with a higher risk of damage to the AV node and should only be considered if well-delivered applications over locations 2, 3, and 5 have not resulted in elimination of 1:1 conduction of the slow pathway.

References

1. Lockwood D, Nakagawa H, Dyer J, Jackman X (2014). Electrophysiological characteristics of atrioventricular nodal reentrant tachycardia: implications for the arrhythmia circuits. In: DP Zipes, J Jalife (eds.). *Cardiac Electrophysiology: From Cell to Bedside*, 3rd edn. Philadelphia: Elsevier Saunders, pp. 767–88.

2. Heidbuchel H. How to ablate typical 'slow/fast' AV nodal reentry tachycardia. *Europace* 2000; **2**: 15–19.

Introduction to the case

A 62-year-old male who presented with palpitations and shortness of breath is shown in Case 64. Six months ago, the patient underwent mitral valve repair, and 2 months ago a typical flutter ablation. An electrophysiological study was undertaken and three catheters (two decapolars and one mapping) were inserted for entrainment mapping in the CS (bipol 9-10 at the os), on the tricuspid ring (RA), and on the cavo-tricuspid isthmus (CTI). During tachycardia with a cycle length of 480ms, the activation on the CS catheter was distal to proximal. The tracing (Figure 64.1) shows the entrainment results from the CS distal (a) and proximal poles (b), the RA catheter (c), and the mapping (CTI) catheter (d).

Figure 64.1 Entrainment results from the CS distal (a) and proximal poles (b), RA catheter (c), and mapping (CTI) catheter (d)

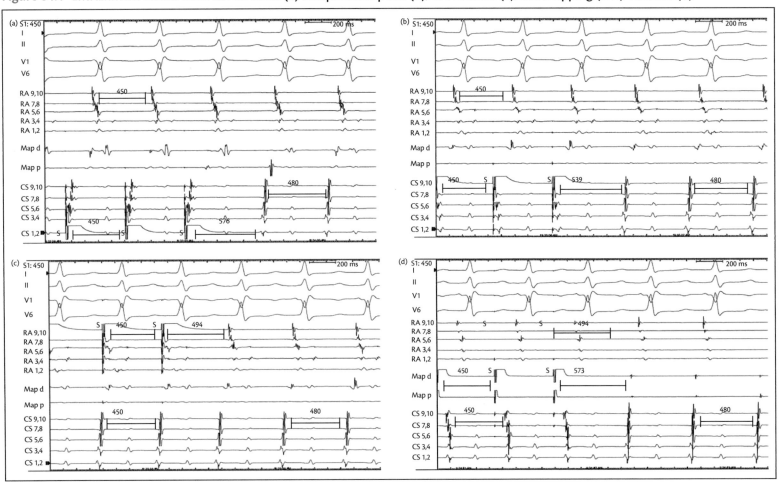

Question

What is the most likely diagnosis of the tachycardia?

A   Left atrial tachycardia

B   CTI-dependent flutter

C   Right atrial free wall tachycardia

D   Focal atrial tachycardia

E   AVRT using a left accessory pathway

Answer

C **Right atrial free wall tachycardia**

Explanation

Entrainment pacing during supraventricular tachycardia

Intracardiac recordings show tachycardia with a cycle length of 480ms, and earliest atrial activation at the distal CS suggests a left atrial circuit.[1] However, entrainment pacing from the distal and proximal CS demonstrated a long PPI, excluding participation of both left atrial sites to the arrhythmia circuit. However, entrainment pacing from the right atrial catheter showed a short difference between the PPI and the TCL (PPI-TCL <30ms) with the same intra-atrial activation sequence during pacing as that during tachycardia, both of which are consistent with a right AT. Entrainment from the CTI revealed a long PPI, excluding isthmus-dependent atrial flutter. It is known that conduction from the right atrium to the left atrium occurs over multiple pathways, including Bachmann's bundle, the foramen ovale, and the CS.[2] Due to block in the CTI as a result of the prior ablation and the presence of a surgical scar in the right atrium, conduction through Bachmann's bundle was more rapid than via the lower septal sites, resulting in distal to proximal left atrial activation, as seen on the CS catheter.

References

1. Pascale P, Shah A, Roten L, *et al.* Pattern and timing of the coronary sinus activation to guide rapid diagnosis of atrial tachycardia after atrial fibrillation ablation. *Circ Arrhythm Electrophysiol* 2013; **6**: 481–90.

2. Roithinger FX, Cheng J, Sippens Groenewegen A, *et al.* Use of electroanatomic mapping to delineate transseptal atrial conduction in humans. *Circulation* 1999; **100**: 1791–7.

Introduction to the case

A 75-year-old male with recurrent AT is referred to in Case 65. There was no previous cardiac surgery or ablations. Recurrence was observed after two successful cardioversions and amiodarone. During tachycardia, the following tracing were recorded during pacing (Figure 65.1) at the (a) proximal CS and (b) distal CS. A schematic representation of right atrium and mapping catheter positions in the LAO projection is also depicted (c).

Figure 65.1 At the (a) proximal CS and (b) distal CS. A schematic representation of right atrium and mapping catheter positions in the LAO projection is also depicted (c). CS1-10: distal to proximal CS; DEC 1-10: anterolateral right atrial wall (see schematic catheters representations in the LAO projection); ⊓: pacing site

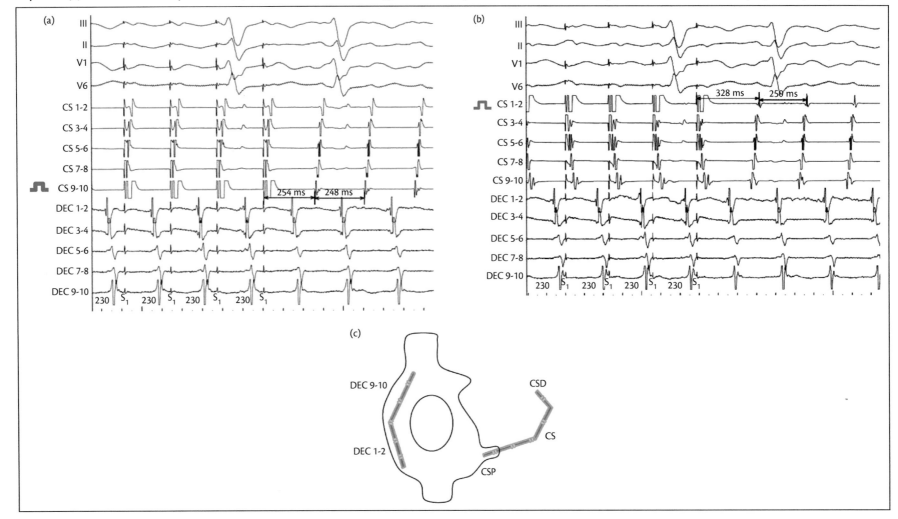

Question

Which of the following is the most likely mechanism of the arrhythmia?

A   Septal macro re-entry

B   'Lower loop' atrial flutter

C   Left atrial re-entry with bystander clockwise right atrial activation

D   Counterclockwise (common) atrial flutter

E   Clockwise (reverse common) atrial flutter

Answer

E   **Clockwise (reverse common) atrial flutter**

Explanation

Entrainment pacing to differentiate intra-atrial re-entrant tachycardia/2

Activation of the right atrium shows caudo-cranial activation f the anterolateral wall of the right atrium, compatible with clockwise progression of the depolarization wavefront.

Entrainment mapping at CS distal excludes a left atrial circuit due to a very long PPI.

Conversely, entrainment from the inferoseptal wall reveals a 'positive' PPI-TCL (i.e. <30ms), confirming that clockwise atrial flutter is the putative mechanism of the tachycardia.

Introduction to the case

Case 66 refers to a 71-year-old male with dilated cardiomyopathy (DCM), LBBB, New York Heart Association (NYHA) class III heart failure, and frequent monomorphic premature ventricular complexes (PVCs). The patient's dual chamber ICD was considered for CRT-D upgrading, but PVCs would preclude optimal biventricular pacing. Radiofrequency ablation (controlled target temperature 55°C, power limit 40W), was attempted at the site of the earliest activity and perfect pacemap (Figure 66.1). After cessation of radiofrequency energy (Figure 66.2, Table 66.1) the PVCs resumed.

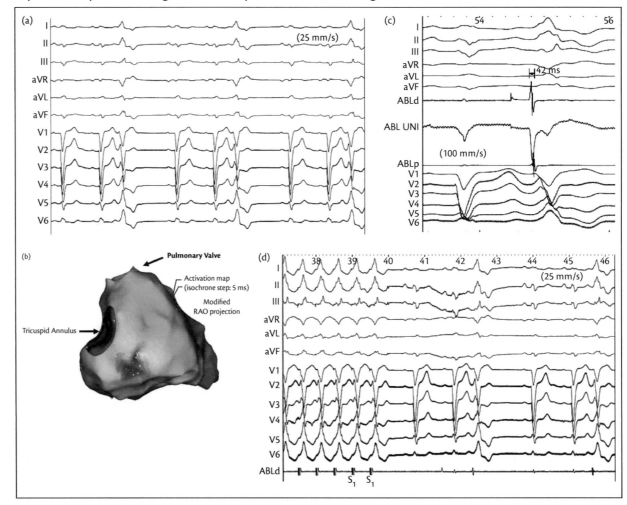

Figure 66.1 PVCs (a) would preclude optimal biventricular pacing rate. Ablation was attempted to overcome the condition. (b) Electro-anatomical mapping confirmed a RV basal free wall origin of ectopics. (c) Site of earliest activation. (d) Pacemap at the site of earliest activation. ABL D: distal bipole of ablation recording; ABL P: proximal bipole recording; ABL UNI: unipolar ablation recording

Figure 66.2 Radiofrequency ablation

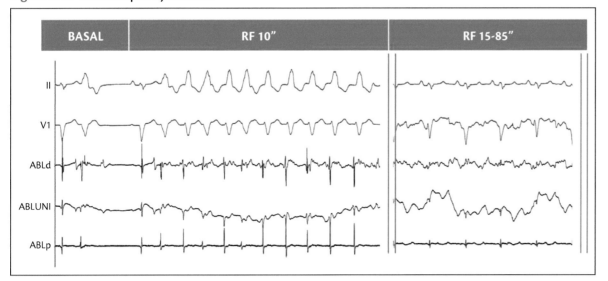

Question

Considering failed ablation, which of the following consideration is right?

A   High likelihood of clinical success due to radiofrequency-induced accelerated VT

B   Ablation with an epicardial approach should be considered

C   A shift towards an open-irrigated catheter should be considered

D   VT induction suggests a re-entrant mechanism; a substrate mapping should be performed before further radiofrequency delivery

E   Despite good pacemap, the ablation site is probably close but not exactly corresponding to the origin of ectopics

Table 66.1 Radiofrequency ablation

	BASAL	RF 10"	RF 15–85"
Impedance (Ω)	126	122	120
Temperature (°C)	37	45	55
Power (W)	-	25	11

Answer

C   A shift towards an open-irrigated catheter should be considered

Explanation

Ablation-resistant premature ventricular complexes

Pacemap, local anticipation of the bipolar electrogram on the surface ECG, and steep QS morphology of the unipolar potential are consistent with the site of origin of the ectopic beats; this is confirmed by immediate induction of accelerated VT early after radiofrequency on-switching.

Ablation is ineffective in this case, most probably due to low power delivery; in fact, radiofrequency parameters are indicating a low-grade impedance drop, along with limited power delivery due to a temperature rise to the maximum cut-off.

RV basal free wall is characterized by low hematic flow and heavy trabeculation; the catheter tip can easily be 'entrapped' and surrounded by tissue, leading to further reduction of blood cooling, generating an excessive temperature rise and consequent power limit.

Although 'irritative' VT during ablation is considered a good predictor of the correct ablation site and of efficacy in the long term, in this case, the result must be considered unsatisfactory, and switching to an open-irrigated catheter should be considered.

In this case, after a change to such a catheter, a single radiofrequency application (power 35W, temperature cut-off 42°C, saline flow 30mL/min) led to immediate cessation of ectopics, and impedance dropped gradually from 120Ω to 98Ω over a 2-minute application with a constant power delivery of 33–35W, resulting in persistent abolition of ventricular ectopic beats (Figure 66.3).[1]

References

1. Baser K, Bas HD, Belardi D, *et al*. Predictors of outcome after catheter ablation of premature ventricular complexes. *J Cardiovasc Electrophysiol* 2014; **2014**: 597–601.

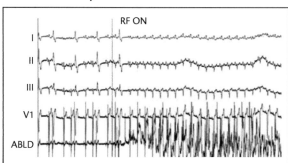

Figure 66.3 A 2-minute application with a constant power delivery of 33–35W, resulting in persistent abolition of ventricular ectopic beats

Introduction to the case

During an electrophysiological study in a woman aged 67 with a long-standing history of paroxysmal SVT, tachycardia is induced by atrial burst pacing. The last two beats of an induction train are shown in Figure 67.1, together with the 1st four beats of tachycardia. Tachycardia episodes always stopped with an atrial electrogram.

Figure 67.1 Induction train. RAA: right atrial appendage; HBp till HBd: His bundle recordings from proximal to distal; PS: posteroseptal recording; CS: coronary sinus; A: atrial electrogram; H: His bundle deflection; S: stimulus

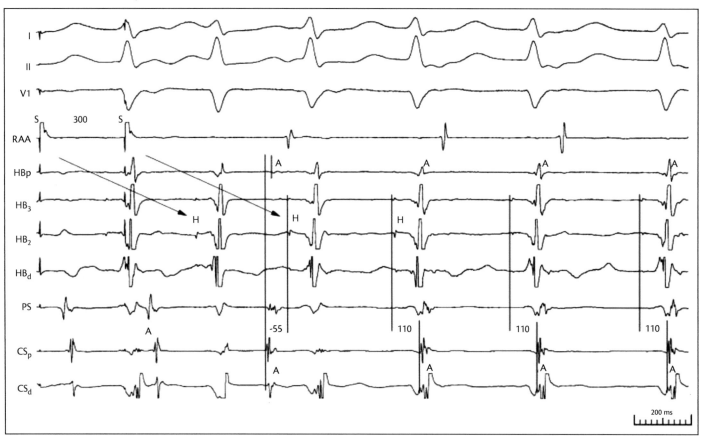

Question

The tracing shows:

A Induction of AT

B Induction of AVRT

C Induction of typical slow/fast AVNRT

D Induction of atypical fast/slow AVNRT

E Induction of atypical slow/slow AVNRT

Answer

E   **Induction of atypical slow/slow AVNRT**

Explanation

An unusual supraventricular tachycardia induction sequence

Rapid atrial pacing results in progressive lengthening of AH intervals at the onset of tachycardia, with an AH interval after the last stimulus of up to 450ms (i.e. the AH interval before the 3rd QRS complex). However, during the 1st tachycardia beat, an unusual pattern occurs of A-before-H, a retrograde atrial activation of the 1st tachycardia beat (A) that precedes the last antegrade His bundle activation (H) by 55ms. The atrial activation sequence reveals the earliest atrial activation in the proximal CS (CSp) and this activation sequence is the same as during the ensuing beats of the tachycardia. In the subsequent beats, atrial activation follows His bundle activation by 110ms.

AT is excluded by the repetitive termination with antegrade block in the AV node.

AVRT is impossible, given the coinciding A and V during tachycardia, and certainly with the A-before-H beat at initiation. The present findings are compatible with slow/slow AVNRT. The negative initial HA interval is the result of delay in the timing of His bundle activation due to a prolonged conduction time through a long LCP. This phenomenon is sometimes present at the initiation of atypical AVNRT (and may oscillate with variable HA intervals during the 1st beats) but is never seen in typical slow/fast AVNRT which has no LCP.[1] The atypical AVNRT in this example is slow/slow AVNRT, since the long AH interval indicates antegrade conduction over the slow pathway.

References

1. Heidbuchel H, Jackman WM. Characterization of subforms of AV nodal reentrant tachycardia. *Europace* 2004; **6**: 316–29.

Introduction to the case

Case 68 discusses a 42-year-old male with a prior ablation for paroxysmal atrial fibrillation. He undergoes a repeat ablation for symptomatic persisting PACs. The Lasso catheter is positioned in the RIPV at the start of the procedure (Figure 68.1).

Figure 68.1 Surface leads II and V1 and intracardiac recordings from the coronary sinus (CS) and Lasso catheter at the left atrium (LA)–PV junction of the right inferior pulmonary vein (RIPV)

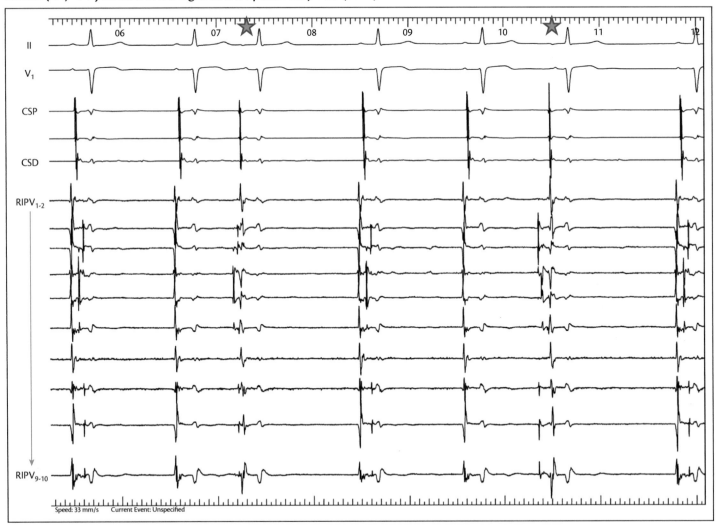

Question

What is the mechanism of the atrial premature beats in this patient?

A   Residual bidirectional conduction at the LA–PV junction of the RIPV

B   Atrial premature beats from the CS ostium

C   Atrial premature beats from the SVC

D   Atrial premature beats from the posterior wall of the left atrium

E   Reconnection of the RSPV

Answer

A   Residual bidirectional conduction at the LA–PV junction of the RIPV

Explanation

Residual bidirectional conduction

The RIPV is characterized by reconnection with residual bidirectional conduction. The 3rd and 6th beats (asterisks) are PACs. The underlying mechanism for the PAC is exit conduction from spontaneous PV beats within the RIPV. These PV beats arise after a specific sequence—the 1st sinus beat is conducted to the RIPV (recording of far-field together with local delayed PV potential); the 2nd sinus beat is blocked at the LA–PV junction (2:1 block) with recording of far-field only (typically from the posterior left atrium in the RIPV). After entry block at the LA–PV junction, a spontaneous PV beat arises (with a different activation pattern of the PV sleeves, compared to entry conduction) which conducts to the left atrium (reversal of activation, i.e. PV potential followed by far-field) and conducts to the ventricle (conducted atrial premature beat with a negative P-wave in lead II and more upright P-wave in V1). After this PAC, the sequence of LA–PV entry conduction, LA–PV entry block, and spontaneous PV beat with exit conduction is repeated. This spontaneous PV beat again is characterized by a manifest different activation pattern of the PV sleeves (now earliest at $RIPV_{3-4}$). The coupling interval of the spontaneous PV beat determines the difference in prematurity of the PAC (whereas the morphology of the P-wave is identical to the 1st premature beat). After closing the gap near $RIPV_{5-6}$, we obtained complete entry block at the LA–PV junction. PV beats continued to exist within the encircled region, but atrial premature beats were eliminated (exit block). The alternative hypothesis that the PACs were due to a marked conduction delay at the LA–PV junction (in contrast to block) with re-entry and exit conduction is unlikely for three reasons: (1) marked shift in PV activation, especially during the 2nd PAC; (2) lack of continuous electrograms compatible with re-entry; and (3) persistence of PV beats after isolation.

Introduction to the case

This case presents a 72-year-old male patient with a 12-month history of persisting atrial fibrillation. The recorded electrograms after circumferential isolation of the left-sided PVs are shown in Figure 69.1.

Figure 69.1 Electrogram recordings after circumferential isolation of the left-sided PVs. The circular mapping catheter is positioned in the LSPV. Lasso: circular mapping catheter inside the LSPV; Abl: ablation/mapping catheter; CS: coronary sinus catheter

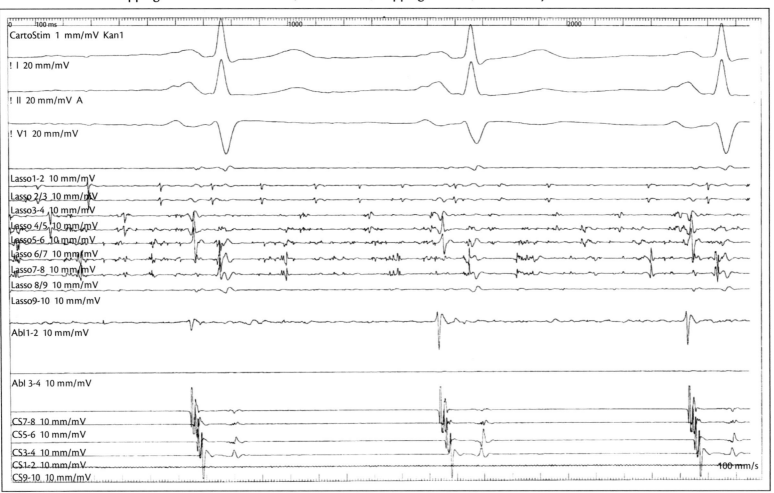

Question

The tracing shows:

A   Ongoing fibrillation of the LSPV, but regular sinus activation of the rest of the atria

B   Noise detection on the Lasso catheter

C   Far-field sensing of atrial fibrillation, but PV isolation

D   Persistent atrial fibrillation

E   Nothing of the above

Answer

A   **Ongoing fibrillation of the LSPV, but regular sinus activation of the rest of the atria.**

Explanation

Dissociated atrial fibrillation within an isolated pulmonary vein

The Lasso catheter positioned in the LSPV shows atrial fibrillation, while surface ECG and CS catheter electrograms indicate stable sinus rhythm.

This indicates at least exit block at the LA–PV junction. Exit block is almost invariably associated with entry block.

Introduction to the case

A girl, aged 15, with manifest pre-excitation on the ECG (indicating a posteroseptal accessory pathway) and paroxysmal palpitations, undergoes an electrophysiological study. An attempt is made to perform para-Hisian pacing from the distal His bundle electrode, but with difficulty to capture. During the attempts, some direct bumps of the His bundle/right bundle branch occur (Figure 70.1).

Figure 70.1 (a) and (b) Direct bumps from the distal His bundle catheter during attempts to pace from it. (c) X-ray of the position of the catheters during recordings. RAA: right atrial appendage; HBE p till HBE d: His bundle recordings from proximal to distal; TA: mapping catheter on the tricuspid annulus; CS: coronary sinus; RAO: right anterior oblique projection; LAO: left anterior oblique projection; red asterisk: site of stimulation

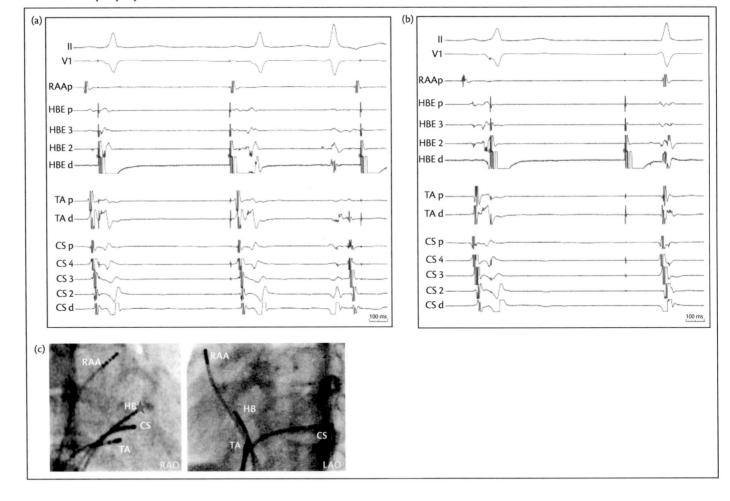

Question

What happens during the His bundle bumps in panels (a) and (b)?

A   These are not bumps, but His bundle automaticity instead.

B   These are not bumps, but retrograde conduction after antegrade Mahaim conduction.

C   Both are associated with retrograde conduction over the accessory pathway.

D   One is associated with retrograde conduction over the AV node, while the other conducts over an accessory pathway.

E   Both are associated with retrograde conduction over the fast AV nodal pathway.

Answer

D **One is associated with retrograde conduction over the AV node, while the other conducts over an accessory pathway.**

Explanation

How catheter bumps can teach us something

His bundle automaticity is excluded because of the clearly different coupling intervals with the foregoing beats. Beats with antegrade conduction over a decrementally conducting accessory pathway ('Mahaim physiology') can result in retrograde right bundle and His bundle activation, but the antegrade conduction over the AV node and His bundle in the foregoing sinus beats, the very long V–H intervals, the variable V–H intervals, and the different atrial retrograde activation sequences all argue against such an explanation.

It is common that during positioning of the His bundle catheter, direct bumps of the His bundle occur. This is associated with a perfectly normal QRS complex, which contrasts with the pre-excited QRS complex in the prior sinus beats (since there is no ventricular capture by the stimulation). The retrograde atrial activation sequence is different, however, in both beats—in the left-sided one, the earliest atrial activation is seen on the posteroseptally located mapping catheter (close to the accessory pathway, as evident from the short A–V during the sinus beats), and the atrial activation at the anterior septum (in the His bundle electrodes) is late. Also, there is a much longer H–A interval than in the right-sided beat (Figure 70.2). The latter shows the earliest atrial activation which is nearly simultaneous in the anterior septum and CS4, while being much later in the mapping catheter (note: right atrial appendage activation may be somewhat shorter than expected, based on retrograde conduction only, and may be explained by fusion with a sinus beat; this, however, has no implications for the interpretation of the tracing). The shorter coupling interval between the last sinus beat and the His bundle bump in panel (a) resulted in a retrograde block in the fast pathway and hence retrograde conduction over the accessory pathway, while in panel (b) (with a much longer coupling interval), there is retrograde conduction over the fast AV nodal pathway. Such conduction is often associated with earliest activation at CS4, via the left side of the atrial septum.

Figure 70.2 further explains the answer.

Figure 70.2 Same tracings at a higher magnification. RAA: right atrial appendage; HBE p till HBE d: His bundle recordings from proximal to distal; TA: mapping catheter on the tricuspid annulus; CS: coronary sinus; RAO: right anterior oblique projection; LAO: left anterior oblique projection; red asterisk: site of stimulation

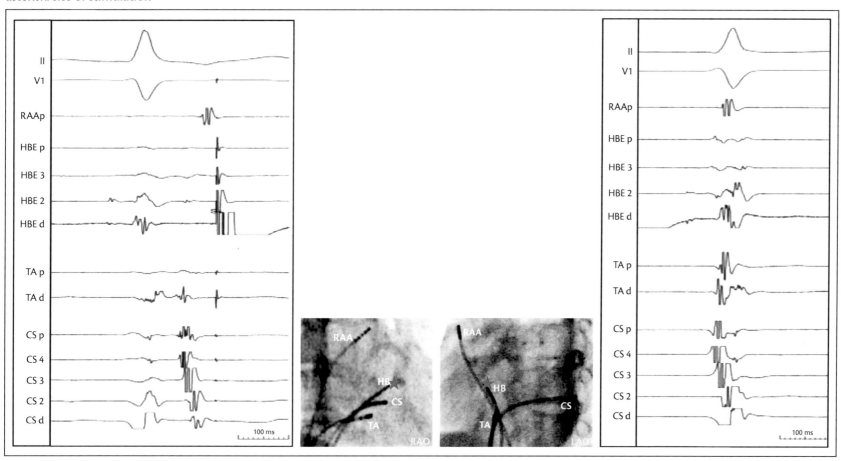

Introduction to the case

A cyclist, aged 27, recorded on his heart rhythm monitor sudden heart rate jumps during exercise, from around 160/min to 220/min, coinciding with symptomatic palpitations and slight dyspnoea. During an electrophysiological study, atrial extrastimuli during isoproterenol administration induced non-sustained episodes of SVT with a cycle length of 280ms, coinciding with jumps in the A–H interval and terminating spontaneously with an antegrade block (Figure 71.1).

Figure 71.1 Episodes of SVT with a cycle length of 280ms. RAA: right atrial appendage; HBp till HBd: His bundle recordings from proximal to distal; A: atrial electrogram; H: His bundle deflection

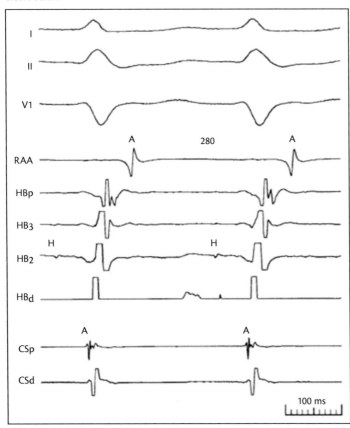

Question

Which form of SVT is present in this patient?

A AVRT over an accessory pathway

B Slow/fast AVNRT

C Fast/slow AVNRT

D Slow/slow AVNRT

E The subform of AVNRT cannot be determined since it is not clear which is the atrial deflection in the His bundle electrograms

Answer

E **The subform of AVNRT cannot be determined since it is not clear which is the atrial deflection in the His bundle electrograms**

Explanation

Differentiating atrioventricular nodal re-entrant tachycardia subforms

AVRT is impossible when retrograde atrial activation is already occurring at the onset of the QRS complex (or if septal VA <70ms, measured from the onset of the surface QRS to septal A). Assuming that AT is ruled out, the tachycardia must be AVNRT.

As often during AVNRT, atrial retrograde activation coincides with ventricular activation. Hence, the site of earliest retrograde atrial activation cannot be determined (it is unclear at this stage whether the terminal deflection on HBp is an atrial potential or a fragmentation of the ventriculogram).

When atrial and ventricular potentials are superimposed, a ventricular extrastimulus delivered to the para-Hisian region through the distal pair of electrodes on the His bundle catheter (HBd), just after antegrade activation of the His bundle, will advance local ventricular, but not atrial, activation (Figure 71.2). This allows distinctive identification of the atrial potential in all electrograms, showing earliest activation in the proximal CS (CSp). Hence, the tachycardia is Slow/Slow AVNRT. This manoeuvre proved that the terminal deflection on the HBp was an atrial potential. Without the ventricular extrastimulus, the tachycardia mimicked slow/fast AVNRT (long A–H interval and short H–A interval). The latter is due to the presence of a long LCP below the turnaround point of the tachycardia in the nodal tissue, which delays anterograde activation of the His (see also Case 5). Earliest atrial activation in the proximal CS indicates retrograde conduction over (a second) slow pathway, excluding typical slow/fast AVNRT, in which earliest atrial retrograde activation is present in the anterior septum close to the His bundle (Figure 71.2).[1]

References

1. Heidbuchel H, Jackman WM. Characterization of subforms of AV nodal reentrant tachycardia. *Europace* 2004; **6**: 316–29.

Figure 71.2 Delivery of a ventricular extrastimulus during tachycardia. RAA: right atrial appendage; HBp till HBd: His bundle recordings from proximal to distal; A: atrial electrogram; H: His bundle deflection

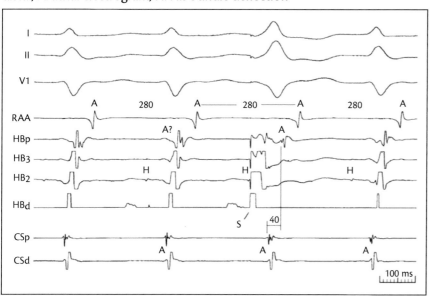

Introduction to the case

The case describes a 64-year-old woman and the evaluation of isolation of the LSPV at the end of the atrial fibrillation ablation procedure (PVI and linear lesions) (Figure 72.1: Pacing distal CS (a), pacing with ablation catheter positioned in LAA (b)).

Figure 72.1 Surface leads II and V1 and intracardiac recordings from the coronary sinus (CS) and Lasso catheter at the LA–PV junction of the left superior pulmonary vein (LSPV); ABLC: ablation catheter; LAA: left atrial appendage

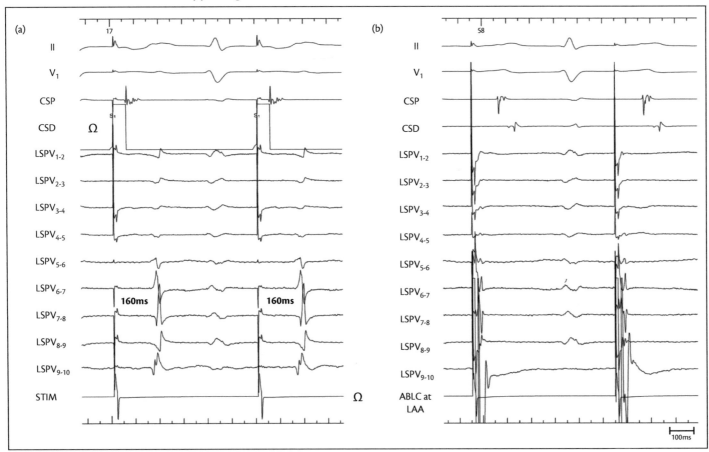

Question

The tracing shows:

A   The LSPV is not isolated (no entry block), and the late atrial potentials (S–A of 160ms) recorded by the Lasso catheter at the LA–PV junction indicate ablation-induced delayed LA–PV conduction

B   The LSPV is characterized by entry block with residual exit conduction

C   The LSPV is isolated, and the late potentials recorded by the Lasso catheter at the LA–PV junction (S–A of 160ms) are far-field recordings of the ventricle

D   The LSPV is isolated, and the late potentials recorded by the Lasso catheter at the LA–PV junction (S–A of 160ms) are far-field recordings of the left atrial appendage in the presence of prior linear ablation

E   The Lasso catheter cannot be in the LSPV

Answer

D **The LSPV is isolated, and the late potentials recorded by the Lasso catheter at the LA–PV junction (S–A of 160ms) are far-field recordings of the left atrial appendage in the presence of prior linear ablation**

Explanation

'Late' far-field from the left atrial appendage

Panel (a): the Lasso was positioned at the LSPV after encircling of the left veins and after linear lesions (roof and mitral isthmus). During regular pacing at the CS (distal bipole), the Lasso recording is characterized by residual atrial potentials (either PV potentials or far-field from the left atrial appendage). The marked delay of 160ms suggests ablation-induced LA–PV delay. Conventionally, however, far-field from the left atrial appendage is picked up within 100ms after the pacing spike during CS pacing.

Panel (b): differential pacing at the left atrial appendage completely 'pulls in' the atrial potentials on the Lasso. This indicates that the residual atrial potentials are far-field recordings from the left atrial appendage. The late left atrial appendage activation during distal CS pacing (160ms) is explained by the presence of block at the mitral isthmus. Block can be appreciated by the proximal to distal activation of the CS during pacing at the left atrial appendage.

Note: the long PR interval is suggestive of prior substrate modification at the septum as well.

Introduction to the case

A 72-year-old patient with a prior inferolateral MI had an ICD implanted for sustained VT. He received multiple shocks, preceded by malaise/syncope, for VTs of different cycle lengths and underwent radiofrequency ablation with substrate modification. An electrogram recorded during mapping of the LV endocardium (during atrial pacing by the ICD at 60 bpm) is shown in Figure 73.1.

Figure 73.1 An electrogram recorded during mapping of the LV endocardium. ABL D: distal ablation; ABL P: proximal ablation; RV: right ventricular apex

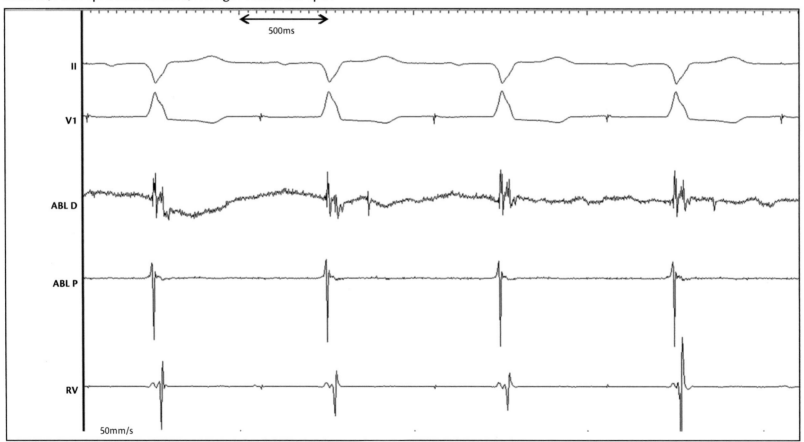

Question

Which of the following statement is false?

A The QRS morphology may be explained by the MI

B A 2:1 late potential is visualized

C Local abnormal ventricular activities (LAVAs) are visible

D The site is certainly part of a re-entry circuit

E This is a suitable site for ablation

Answer

D The site is certainly part of a re-entry circuit

Explanation

Substrate modification for post-myocardial infarction ventricular tachycardia

The CARTO voltage map is shown in Figure 73.2. The left axis deviation and R-wave in lead V1 may be explained by the inferolateral scar (although intraventricular conduction delay is also present due to a QRS duration of 140ms). The electrogram on the ablation catheter was recorded in region of scar. Late potentials indicate slow local conduction and are targets for substrate modification.[1] The 2:1 local conduction of the late potentials, however, make it unlikely that these potentials are a critical part of the re-entrant circuit. The electrogram, however, also shows fractionated and split potentials that are compatible with LAVAs, which may be associated with re-entrant circuits (but this is not for certain) and are also targets for radiofrequency ablation aiming to eliminate these potentials.

References

1. Jais P, Maury P, Khairy P. Elimination of local abnormal ventricular activities. A new end point for substrate modification in patients with scar-related ventricular tachycardia. *Circulation* 2012; **125**: 2184–96.

Figure 73.2 The CARTO voltage map

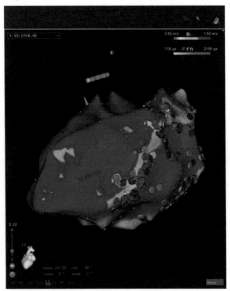

Introduction to the case

Because of an unclear entrance block of the LSPV, this pacing is performed from the 10-pole Lasso catheter positioned within the encircled PV (distal to the ablation site) (Figure 74.1). Pacing is performed at Lasso bipole A4 with high and low output.

Figure 74.1 Pacing is performed at Lasso bipole A4 with high and low output. A: bipolar electrograms from the 10-pole ablation catheter; CS: coronary sinus catheter

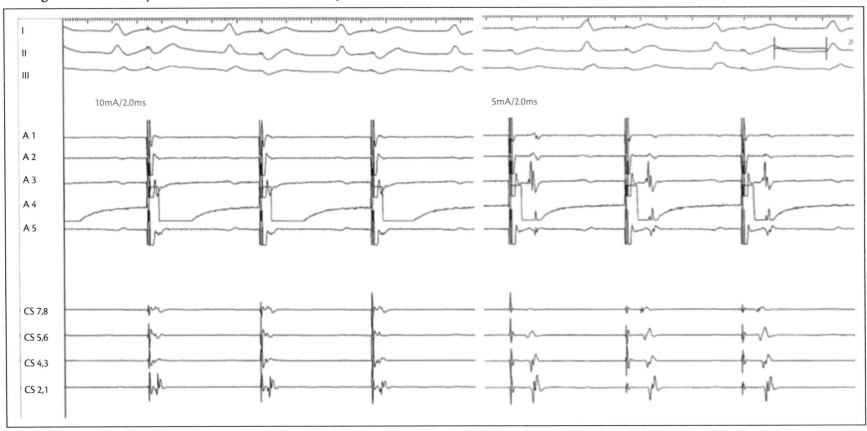

Question

The pacing manoeuvre indicates residual exit conduction based on the finding that:

A   High- and low-output PV pacing produces no capture

B   High- and low-output PV pacing shows far-field capture but no PV capture

C   Low-output exit pacing shows a 1:1 relation to the CS

D   Only low-output pacing provides far-field capture

E   Low-output pacing shows no conduction to the left atrium

Answer

C   **Low-output exit pacing shows a 1:1 relation to the CS**

Explanation

Pulmonary vein exit block testing with residual conduction

High-output PV pacing (10mA/2.0ms) leads to far-field capture of left atrial tissue (short conduction time to CS 1/2), which makes evaluation of exit conduction impossible.

With lower pacing output (5mA/2.0ms), the delay in conduction time to CS 1/2 indicates a shift to near-field PV capture only. This manoeuvre shows residual exit conduction (no exit block). The finding of exit conduction in the presence of 'unclear' entrance block makes the diagnosis of residual entry conduction very likely.

Introduction to the case

This case describes a 66-year-old woman who was implanted with a CRT-D and recording a regular wide QRS tachycardia (175 bpm) (Figure 75.1).

Figure 75.1 Recording of a regular wide QRS tachycardia. Surface leads V1 and intracardiac recordings from the proximal and distal bipoles of the His bundle (HB) and right ventricular apex (RVA)

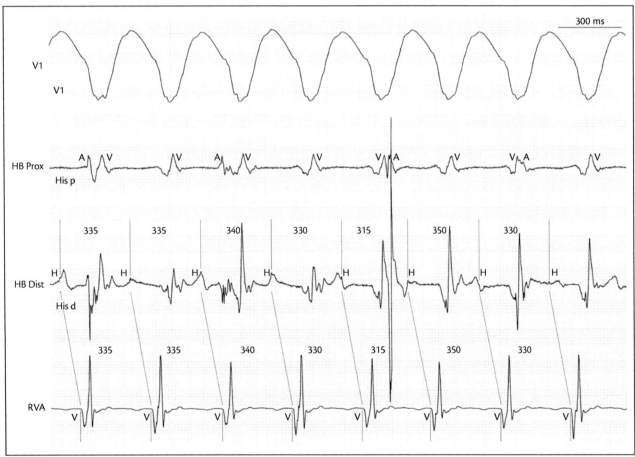

Question

The mechanism of tachycardia is:

A AVNRT in the presence of pre-existing LBBB

B Orthodromic AVRT via the nodo-fascicular pathway

C Pre-excited tachycardia

D BBRVT

E AT in the presence of pre-existing LBBB

Answer

D **BBRVT**

Explanation

Bundle branch re-entrant ventricular tachycardia

BBRVT was diagnosed based upon the following findings on the intracardiac bipolar electrograms: (1) AV dissociation (atrial activation can be detected on the proximal recording of the His bundle catheter); (2) His deflections present 102ms before the onset of each QRS (during sinus rhythm, the HV interval was already prolonged at 72ms; not shown); and (3) cycle length oscillations (315–350ms) with changes in the HH interval preceding changes in the VV interval. Catheter ablation was performed with a 4-mm non-irrigated tip catheter and consisted of radiofrequency ablation of the right bundle branch during sinus rhythm.

Introduction to the case

Case 76 shows a 20-year-old woman with palpitations. Transition from a 2:1 narrow complex tachycardia to a 1:1 wide complex tachycardia is shown in Figure 76.1.

Figure 76.1 Transition from a 2:1 narrow complex tachycardia to a 1:1 wide complex tachycardia. Surface leads II and V1 and intracardiac recordings from the high right atrium (HRA), His bundle (HB), coronary sinus (CS), and right ventricular apex (RVA)

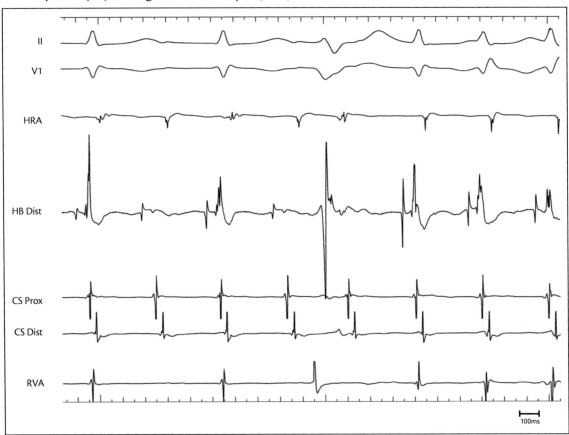

Question

What is the mechanism of transition?

A   SVT with a spontaneous PVC inducing VT

B   Atrial flutter inducing AVNRT

C   AVNRT with resumption of 1:1 infra-Hisian conduction after a PVC

D   AVNRT with resumption of 1:1 conduction over the LCP after a PVC

E   Atypical AVNRT inducing atrial flutter

Answer

C **AVNRT with resumption of 1:1 infra-Hisian conduction after a PVC**

Explanation

Slow/fast atrioventricular nodal re-entrant tachycardia and infra-Hisian block

Figure 76.1 (left): 2:1 tachycardia compatible with AVNRT or AT (cycle length of 286ms). Orthodromic AVRT and VT are excluded. There is 2:1 infra-Hisian AV block. A His bundle potential is recorded in the blocked complexes.

Figure 76.1 (middle): a spontaneous premature ventricular beat from the RV with early precocity advances His and atrial activation. Advancement of atrial activation by a PVC occurs in AVRT, but also in cases of early precocity in AVNRT and AT. The PVC unmasks the atrium at the His bundle electrogram (after the retrograde H deflection). The earliest A at the His bundle electrogram (anterior septum) suggests slow/fast AVNRT. In slow/fast AVNRT, 2:1 AV block is due to infra-Hisian block (absence of LCP) and maintained by long refractoriness at the proximal His–Purkinje system (prolonged refractoriness is explained by the 2-fold longer cycle length just distal from the site block).

Figure 76.1 (right): the PVC results in early retrograde activation of the His bundle. Together with delayed conduction over the slow pathway, this lengthens the H–H interval, enabling resumption of 1:1 AV conduction. Because of a prolonged A–H interval over the slow pathway, the cycle length is prolonged during the next AVNRT beats (cycle length of 298ms). This facilitates 1:1 infra-Hisian AV conduction (longer H–H interval), now with block in the right bundle (whereas before there was block in both bundles).

After ablation of the slow pathway, the tachycardia was rendered non-inducible.

Index